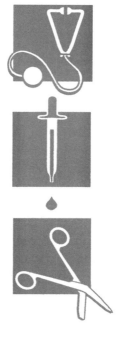

The
Basics of
Camp
Nursing

Linda Ebner Erceg
RN, MS, PHN

Myra Pravda
RN, MSN

American Camping Association®

Copyright 2001 by American Camping Association, Inc.

Printed in the United States of America

All rights reserved. No part of this book may be reproduced or transmitted in any form or by any means, electronic or mechanical, including photocopying, recording, or any information storage retrieval system, without permission in writing from the publisher.

Cover photo by Aire Steinberg, Los Angeles, California.

All product and company names mentioned herein are the trademarks of their respective owners.

American Camping Association, Inc.
5000 State Road 67 North
Martinsville, IN 46151-7902
765-342-8456   national office
800-428-2267   bookstore
765-349-6357   fax
bookstore@ACAcamps.org   e-mail
www.ACAcamps.org   web site

Library of Congress Cataloging-in-Publication Data

Erceg, Linda Ebner, 1949-
    The basics of camp nursing / Linda Ebner Erceg, Myra Pravda.
        p. ; cm.
    Includes bibliographical references and index.
    ISBN 0-87603-173-4
        1. Camp nursing. I. Pravda, Myra, 1941 - II. American
    Camping Association III. Title.
    [DNLM: 1. Nursing Care—United States. 2. Camping—United
    States. WY 100 E65b 2001]
    RT120.C3 E73 2001
    610.73—dc21

                                                          2001034119

. . . To our husbands, Marv and David, for their support and patience.

. . . To our children — Andrea, Elaina, Joel, and Laura — who loved camp and grew up there.

. . . To our camps — Camp Livingston, the Cincinnati JCC Day Camp, Camp Chinqueka, and the Concordia Language Villages — for giving us the opportunity to be their camp nurses.

Contents

Chapter 5

Chapter 6

Chapter 12

Chapter 13

References and Resources

Appendix

Preface

The Basics of Camp Nursing provides an overview of a camp nurse's role. Typical practices and policies are described with the understanding that the philosophy of an individual camp will color the way this information is used. In addition, regulatory bodies influence nursing practice as well as camp practices. For these reasons, contents of this book should be interpreted and applied with respect to:

- The Nurse Practice Act of the state in which the camp is located and, therefore, the state in which the camp nurse should be licenced
- The Association of Camp Nurses' Standards of Camp Nursing Practice
- The entity from which the camp is licenced to operate
- The American Camping Association's *Accreditation Standards for Camp Programs and Services*
- The American Nurses Association Standards of Nursing Practice
- The insurances held by the camp
- The camp's administrative directives, policy statements, job descriptions, and other reliable sources of information

The Basics of Camp Nursing was written for use by registered nurses (RN) and uses the word "nurse" in reference to an RN. It is not intended to guide the practice of Licensed Practical Nurses who often have a supervision component which must be fulfilled in order to practice as nurses. The book addresses needs of the entry-level camp nurse, a novice in camp practice. Suggested practices are exactly that — suggested. It is incumbent upon you to thoughtfully consider the ramifications of actions as they pertain to the situation of the moment; follow best practice guidelines. Above all, do no harm.

Abbreviations and Definitions

ABCD	Airway, Breathing, Circulation, Deformity (Primary Assessment)
ACA	American Camping Association
ACN	Association of Camp Nurses
AD/HD	Attention deficit hyperactivity disorder
ADL	Activities of daily living
APAP	Acetaminophen
AR	Artificial respiration
ASA	Aspirin
ASAP	As soon as possible
AVPU	Alert, Verbal, Pain, Unconscious
BID	Twice a day
BM	Bowel movement
bndg	Bandage, band-aid
BS	Bowel sounds
CCI	Christian Camping International
CMS	Color, Movement, Sensation
CPR	Cardio-pulmonary respiration
DM	Diabetes mellitus
DMR	Daily medication record
Dx	Diagnosis
EMS	Emergency response system
FA	First Aid
GI	Gastro-intestinal
HA	Healthcare assistant
HAS	Health and safety coordinator
HC	Health center
LOC	Level of consciousness
MOI	Mechanism of injury
MSDS	Material safety data sheet
OTC	Over-the-counter (medications)
PCA	Personal care attendant

PDR	Physician's desk reference
PEARL	Pupils equal and reactive to light
PPE	Personal protective equipment
prn	As needed
q	Every
qD	Every day
QID	Four times a day
Rx	Prescription
S/S	Signs/symptoms
TAO	Triple antibiotic ointment
TID	Three times a day
Tx	Treatment
URI	Upper respiratory infection
WF	Waterfront

Health Form — A form, provided by the camp to staff and campers, which is completed within six months of camp arrival and which focuses on a given individual's health history. Two elements, a physician's exam and parental permission to treat, are often part of the health form.

Health Log — Published by ACA, this bound book with numbered pages provides a way to list the names of people seen for health care chronologically; each page is dated. Used to quickly know who was seen in the health center on a given day and for what purpose.

Health Record(s) — Documentation about the health care given to specific individuals while at camp. Format varies from camp to camp.

Personal Medications — Medications brought by an individual camper or staff member and used to meet personal health needs under the direction of a personal physician.

Screening — A process of reviewing the health status of campers and staff within twenty-four hours of arrival. The elements of screening vary based on the nature of the camp program and the health status of clients who attend.

Stock Medications — Medications provided by the camp, used by the nurse, and supported by medical protocols.

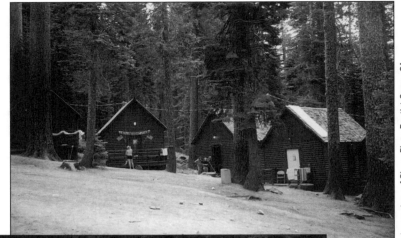

Photo courtesy of Sierra Pines Baptist Camp, CA

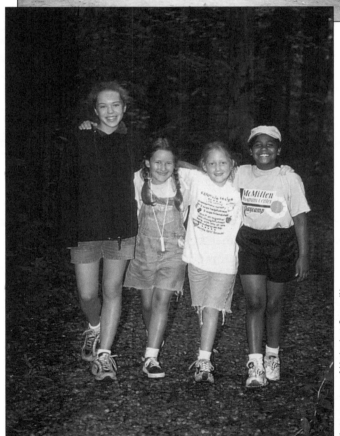

Photo courtesy of Limberlost Camp, IN

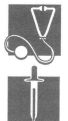

CHAPTER 1

The Nurse at Camp

Camp is a unique and challenging practice setting for nurses. It is very different from working in a hospital, nursing home, physician's office, or school. It's an opportunity to work with children, youth, and other adults in a child-centered outdoor environment. It's a job that calls for a variety of nursing skills but it's also one for which nurses often feel unprepared. Camp nursing courses are rare and access to educational material about camp nursing is limited. The purpose of this book is to change some of that. Building on your basic nursing knowledge, you'll discover the world of camp nursing described in camp terminology along with familiar nursing language. A bit of humor occasionally peppers comments because camp, at its heart, is fun.

Today's camp nurse provides day-to-day health care to campers and camp staff, maintains health records, administers medication, manages the health center, responds to emergencies, collaborates with out-of-camp resources, and communicates with staff and parents. In addition, the nurse is a health educator, risk manager, and sanitarian. Being at camp — which entails, for many camp nurses, actually living there — means the nurse is highly visible and accessible to both campers and staff. The camp nurse is a vital part of today's camp community.

This wasn't always so. Camp nursing has only recently started to emerge as a practice specialty with a community health focus. Prior to the 1990s, many camps had "infirmaries" where nurses stayed and took care of injuries and illnesses. The nurse was a support staff person; rarely did she or he contribute to the camp program or leave the infirmary.

Today the camp nurse is a professional whose commitment to care — the heart of nursing practice — is valued by camp administration, camp parents, and the staff and campers with whom the nurse interacts. Infirmaries are fast giving way to health centers, and nurses are building a repertoire of resources by working with one another to improve the health of people at camp. Mere treatment no longer suffices; prevention of injury and illness matters. The concept of "health services" has been introduced (Erceg, 1999a; Erceg, 1999b) and *The Standards and Scope of Camp Nursing Practice* is available (Association of Camp Nurses, 2001).

The Camp Setting — the Camp Nurse's Environment

Basically, there are two types of camps: residential and day camps. In a resident facility the campers and staff live at the camp and stay for a period of time. The environment can range from urban to a remote wilderness setting. A resident camp session can be anywhere from three days to eight weeks in length. Day campers and staff, on the other hand, come to camp in the morning and return to their homes in the afternoon. Camps may be single gender or coed. The number of campers varies from as few as twenty-five campers in a small program to very large camps with hundreds of campers.

The American Camping Association (2001) estimates that there are 8,500 to 10,000 camps nationwide with more than 9 million youth benefiting from a summer camp experience. The number of day camps in the United States is estimated at 3,000. The approximately 900,000 camp jobs are filled each summer by college students, teachers, nurses, doctors, and many others who wish to make a positive difference in the lives of the campers.

Camps can be privately owned, have an agency affiliation (e.g., YMCA, Girl Scouts, Boy Scouts, Easter Seals) or a church affiliation.

16

A privately owned camp may be a sole proprietorship or there may be several owners who have formed a camp corporation. A board may be the decision-making body for agency- and church-affiliated camps, whereas a single person — the camp owner — may be the decision maker at a different camp. It is important for the camp nurse to know who operates the camp because these individuals make decisions about camp policy and the nurse is usually accountable to them.

Some camps utilize school or community buildings and take the campers to nearby parks and swimming pools. Other camps have their own buildings but may be in extremely remote areas. The camp's location is important for accessing emergency and other community resources. Also, the physical environment of the camp impacts the health needs of the participants. A wilderness camp with no running water or electricity requires a different health care approach from that of a camp with running water and electricity which is also within fifteen minutes of a trauma center.

Camps, especially resident camps, operate as small communities. Staff and campers usually stay in or, in the case of day camps, gather together in cabins or bunks. These cabins or bunks often form units that are generally sensitive to the age of campers. These units, the counseling staff working in them, and kitchen, maintenance, program, health, and administrative staff make up the camp community. All these individuals work together to make the camp function effectively.

Camp programs — what campers do — vary. Camps offering a "general program" provide a variety of activities such as arts and crafts, aquatics, sports, drama, archery, and horseback riding. Specialty camps offer concentration in such areas as soccer, computers, music, language, or travel. Some camps offer programs in self-improvement (academic tutoring or programs for the gifted, for example). Other camps, often called "special needs camps," work with clients who share a particular health focus such as cancer, diabetes, arthritis, behavioral problems, weight management, or spina bifida. There are even camps serving children who are ventilator dependent.

Summer camps primarily have children in attendance. The camp environment is unique and nurturing, yet fosters independence for participants. It is a wonderful setting for children to gain confidence, overcome fears, and develop self-reliance. Campers learn new skills in an outdoor environment and are encouraged to use their creativity while independent from their family. Camp friendships — for staff as well as campers — often last a lifetime.

Camp Staff

The staff comprises all the people who work at camp. Staff positions may be either paid or volunteer. The camp nurse typically has some responsibilities related to staff health.

Typically, summer staff are seasonal employees who work the entire camp season, although this isn't always the case. Camp staff, hired by the camp director, start their summer with staff orientation (also called "precamp"). Those with program responsibilities are often specialists in an area such as the waterfront, crafts, horseback riding, or sports. Counseling staff, on the other hand, focus on the campers and are usually supervised by a unit head, team leader, or head counselor. Some camps combine these roles; counselors have both cabin and activity responsibilities. Cabin groups are generally made up of at least two counselors and a group of between eight and ten campers who are the same age and gender. The camp nurse probably works most closely with the counseling staff to meet the needs of campers, but also interfaces with other staff to address broad, community health needs.

Camping Organizations

The Association of Camp Nurses (ACN) is a professional nursing organization established to promote and develop nursing practice in the camp community. This volunteer organization is driven by nurses who are committed to promoting healthy camp communities. ACN's Web site (www.campnurse.org) makes access to membership, the Camp Nurse Store, conferences, workshops, and other support only a click away. ACN also provides *The Standards and Scope of Camp Nursing Practice* (2001).

The American Camping Association (ACA) is an organization of camp professionals dedicated to enriching children and adult lives through the camp experience. ACA has developed *Standards* for camp accreditation (American Camping Association, 1998). These *Standards*, while voluntary in nature, focus on basic safety and good business practices. Some camps choose to be ACA accredited; this means that the camp is visited once every three years by a team of ACA volunteers who assess the camp's compliance with the *Standards*. Assuming successful completion of the *Standards*, the camp is accredited. You will find ACA's Web site very informative (www.ACAcamps.org).

Christian Camping International/USA (CCI/USA) is an international alliance of Christian Camping Associations helping one another in the development of Christian camps, conferences, and retreat ministries. CCI/USA, found online at www.cci.org, holds conferences, follows ACA Standards, and includes nursing in their risk management section.

Acquiring a Camp Nurse Position

Camp nurse positions are advertised in local newspapers, nursing journals, and online through ACN's as well as other nursing job sites. Advertisements begin to appear in early winter and continue until camp nurse positions are filled. Sometimes a nurse doesn't even consider camp as a practice option until her or his own child reaches camp age. That's the point at which sources that help parents find a camp — e.g., the *ACA Guide to Accredited Camps*, *Frost's Summer Camp Guide*, *Peterson's Guide to Camps*, and many Web sites — may trigger interest from the parent who is also a nurse.

Camps have literature about their camp programs. When contacting a camp, ask for this printed material as well as the camp video. Visit the camp's Web site. These sources provide interested nurses with a great overview of the camp.

When interviewing for a camp nurse position, ask for:

- A copy of the camp's job description for the nurse.
- A description of the work day. Is the nurse in the setting twenty-four hours a day? The camp might have one nurse who functions in an autonomous role or several nurses who rotate shifts in the health center.

- An indication of time off. Who covers for the nurse during this time?
- A description of the staff and campers. How many of each are there? Where do they come from? Are they from the state or does the camp draw from many states? Are campers primarily inner city, suburban, or rural?
- A description (or photo) of the health center and the nurse's living quarters.
- The camp's policy about family members at camp. Can the nurse's children be campers? How is a spouse's visit handled?
- A description of a typical day from the nurse's perspective (not what the camp is doing but what the nurse does).
- The salary and benefits.
- The policy on reimbursing licensing fees.

Nursing License

To practice as a nurse, you must be licensed by the state in which the camp is located. Contact the state's board of nursing for information about getting a license. Apply as soon as possible. Some states move licensing requests quickly while others drag out the process.

Professional Liability Insurance

Camps usually carry liability insurance. Talk with the camp director about the camp's position in case of a lawsuit involving the camp nurse. If something were to happen, the camp's lawyer generally would act in the best interest of the camp; this may not be in the nurse's best interest. Ultimately you will need to balance your professional liability, the camp's position, and your need for insurance while at camp. Some homeowner's policies will attach a rider that provides this insurance for a nominal fee. Inquire about it before starting the job.

CHAPTER 2

Before Going to Camp

Review These Materials

Camp health needs vary and are influenced by the camp population, the type of program offered, the length of camp sessions, the number of health care providers on site, the distance to emergency services, and the availability of community resources. These elements affect the written policies for a camp's health services program. Ask to read the camp's **Healthcare Plan** (ACA Standard HW-3). It often describes the needs of the campers and staff and how these needs should be met. In other words, it may describe the scope of healthcare provided by the camp. It may also describe the counseling staff's responsibility regarding camp health care and the medical, mental health, dental, and pharmaceutical resources of the local community. The plan may also specify the policies and procedures for healthcare staff. ACA-accredited camps are asked to formally review their health polices and procedures every three years (ACA Standard HW-4) and update them annually.

In addition to the camp's Healthcare Plan, be sure to read

- Information specific to the camp's health center: the policies and procedures manual, the camp's Exposure Control Plan, a list of stocked medications and supplies, and the physician's treatment protocols.

- A copy of the camper and staff health form(s). (See p. 82.)
- A copy of the staff manual (one from the year before is adequate). This manual explains how the camp operates, its history and philosophy, the general responsibilities of staff, and the personnel policies. It may also discuss what to bring to camp, counseling tips, camper information, rules that are followed, camp programming areas, dining hall procedures, general health information, transportation, and emergency procedures.
- A schedule of a typical camp day; ask how the nurse's schedule interfaces.
- The previous summer's health logs and/or camper and staff health records. A summary of injury and illness patterns for the past few years may be available.
- A staff orientation schedule. (The nurse is usually responsible for a health presentation during orientation; is that the case for this camp?)
- A copy of regulations that impact health services for the camp (e.g., state health regulations, ACA Standards).
- *The Standards and Scope of Camp Nursing Practice* (Association of Camp Nurses, 2001).
- The Nurse Practice Act from the state in which the camp is located.

Talk with the Camp Director

Both the camp director and you will have expectations regarding the nurse's role at camp. Some expectations may be based on camp tradition while others may be tied to policy. Some reflect the way the director would like the camp to function and others reflect how you perceive the job. Regardless of etiology, you and the director should have common expectations. Work toward this goal by talking with the camp director about the following:

1. How is the nurse's role viewed in the camp culture? Are people used to the nurse staying in the health center (all the time) or does the nurse get out and about camp to talk with people about health and safety concerns? Will your approach to the job alter the camp's expectation of the nurse?
2. Is the nurse part of the camp's core staff or ancillary to the camp?

22

3. Does the nurse have a role at staff meetings and do staff consult with her or him when activities they plan impact people's health and/or safety?
4. Where does the nurse fit into the organizational chart of the camp?
5. Are there former camp nurses that you can contact to learn about the camp and the nursing functions there?
6. When things get busy in the health center, who helps? What are their qualifications? Is there a job description for this role? Is this assistance scheduled by the camp director or the nurse? If the nurse is expected to delegate responsibility, discuss the tasks that can be delegated and how those tasks might be monitored.
7. Who is the camp physician? What's the experience of the camp with this doctor?
8. When and how should the director and nurse communicate with one another? Will the director stop in the health center to review the log to find out how things are going, or is the expectation that the nurse will tell the director when there's something of interest to report? Does this plan make sense for this summer?
9. How is the nurse evaluated? Is a job performance tool used?
10. If the camp director could select one area of health to improve during the summer, what would that be? Discuss how to accomplish that improvement.
11. Finally, ask the camp director: "What do you think I need to help me succeed as your camp's nurse?"

Brush Up on Clinical Skills

Campers and staff come to camp with chronic illnesses, special needs, on daily medication, and following special dietary needs. At most camps, campers have completed a health form which is sent to camp before the camp session begins. The information on these forms provides the nurse with a glimpse of anticipated clinical needs. They also contain emergency contact information and have been signed by parents or guardians giving the camp permission to treat the child for illness and injury.

Consider brushing up on clinical skills by visiting a pediatrician, a family practice physician, and/or a dentist. Go to a local ambulance service, explain that you're going to camp, and ask them to explain their response process. Also consider:

1. Getting current certification in first aid and CPR. Consider taking a wilderness first aid course if at all possible — the critical decision-making skills make this worth the investment.
2. Taking a Camp Nurse Workshop (see ACN's Web site for current list).
3. Reading other camp nursing literature (see ACN's Web site under "References and Resources").
4. Building clinical skill in the following areas:
   a. Using an otoscope, doing an ear exam, recognizing visualized landmarks within the ear.
   b. With regard to asthma management, knowing:
      • How and when to use a peak flow meter.
      • How a nebulizer works, what it does, and what medication(s) is commonly nebulized.
   c. Knowing how to test blood sugar using a lancet with visual strip checking.
   d. Assessing a sore throat.
   e. Handling minor orthodontic repairs such as removing a loose bracket, reattaching an elastic, and knowing when *not* to cut a wire.
   f. Backboarding.
   g. Recognizing and managing anaphylaxis in the field.
   h. Assessing injuries to joints (ankles, knees, shoulders) and sports injuries.
5. Reviewing medications commonly used in the pediatric and youth population. Pay special attention to
   a. Asthma medications.
   b. Psychotropic medications, especially those used for AD/HD.
   c. Allergy medications.

Finally, consider reading Crane's article, "Five Rookie Mistakes and Five Lessons Learned" (2000). This light read puts camp into perspective and draws attention to the fact that camp is fun. Don't get so carried away with what might happen that you lose sight of all the fun you're going to have.

CHAPTER 3

Camp Nurse Tasks During Staff Orientation (Precamp)

Things done by the camp nurse prior to the arrival of campers.

Some camp nurses do not attend staff orientation; they work later in the season and, as a result, miss the discussions, problem-solving, and skills addressed during staff orientation. Nonetheless, no matter when during the season a nurse may work, he or she needs to know the information is this section because it sets the tone for the camp's expectations from health services. Outgoing camp nurses can pass the information to incoming nurses. Be sure to do this!

Health Service Defined

The camp nurse collaborates with the camp director to provide the camp's health services. Talk with the director about his or her expectations of the healthcare staff. Some of the topics listed below help create an interface between the camp program (what counselors and campers do) and the nurse's responsibilities. Items to discuss include:

1. The camp policy regarding cabin and sanitation check (referred to as the Nurse's Walk-around): Who is responsible for checking? What is checked?
2. Time and content of the health orientation for the camp staff; in particular, ask to see any written procedures (refer to the next section, "Health Orientation for Camp Staff," and to ACA Standard HW-12).

3. The time during orientation when staff screening should be conducted (see Appendix B).
4. The camp nurse's role in nonmedical emergencies (e.g., threatening weather or a missing camper).
5. Health center management:
   a. What are the health center's office hours?
   b. How and when are medications dispensed?
   c. How is the health center secured and who has access?
   d. Who needs to know when the nurse calls a camper's parent and/or the camp's physician, clinic, hospital, dentist, etc.?
   e. Who does the nurse tell when a camper is admitted to the health center? When a counselor is admitted?
6. Doctor appointments:
   a. How do people get to appointments? Who takes them?
   b. Who accompanies campers? What information does the director need afterward?
   c. If a prescription is needed, where is it filled? Who pays for it?
7. Who provides healthcare when the nurse is unavailable and during scheduled time off? When does this person come for training?
8. How are health center requests for repair and maintenance routed?
9. What is the procedure for communicating with the director and staff about health and safety issues during the camp season?
10. When does the nurse talk with campers to orient them to the camp's health service (refer to "Health Talk to Campers")?
11. Who helps at the health center and what is their role?
12. About what issues does the director expect to be informed?

Practice Hint

This is the place to discuss confidentiality, the camp's mandated reporting process, and who has access to what information about camper and staff health.

13. Who has the responsibility for notifying parents in an emergency as well as for routine health concerns. Who places these calls and

who needs to be informed? What has the camp told parents about notification? (See ACA Standard HW-17.)

14. The camp's OSHA programs, in particular the camp's exposure control plan. Who is responsible for educating staff about this information?

15. Some state regulations may be restrictive about campers arriving at camp with medications. Some require the medication to arrive in its original package with appropriate labeling in place. Ask about your state regulations and what parents have been told about sending medication with the camper.

Health Orientation for Camp Staff

The purpose of this talk is to acquaint personnel with the camp's health center program. Note that several topics are suggested and there may not be time to do everything. In fact, camp directors often predetermine time allocated for the nurse's talk when they plan staff orientation, so be prepared to be succinct. Consider prioritizing information based on the needs of staff and using other staff meetings to cover items that don't get fully explained.

The objective of the talk is to describe the staff's role in maintaining their own health and that of the campers so boundaries are clear. In so doing, point out areas in which harm could be done (e.g., attempting to be their cabin's doctor).

In addition to providing staff with health-specific information, recognize that while leading this orientation session, you are communicating your "camp competence," and the staff is assessing:

- How approachable is this nurse? Would I want to discuss a concern with him or her?
- How caring is this nurse? Will the nurse see me or the campers as a person or just the illness or injury that we present?
- How knowledgeable is the nurse? Does the nurse have a basic understanding of camp's impact on health and is she or he willing to get help from others when personal knowledge just isn't enough?

Consequently, take time to adequately prepare and consider how you want to deliver information (lecture, series of questions, etc.). It is also a good idea to tell the staff how you came to be at camp and share your camp background as well as your nursing experience. An organized, informative session with staff is a critical step in addressing the questions they have about you.

Items to consider including during the staff orientation talk are:

1. Information about health center routine, especially office hours; when and how medications are dispensed; and the availability of out-of-camp providers. Emphasize that the health center is a resource for everyone at camp — staff included.
2. Cabin and sanitation inspection procedures (a.k.a. the Nurse's Walk-around).
3. What staff should do about their own health concerns:
   a. Turning in health forms with complete information.
   b. Giving all personal medication to the health center staff.
   c. Reporting their own illness/injury even when minor to avoid major complications.
4. Describe camper health-related issues that counselors can help with.
   a. Helping campers maintain personal cleanliness and hygiene.
   b. Formulating strategies for coping with the lack of privacy.
   c. Noting signs of illness and sensing when to bring ill campers to the nurse.
   d. Coaching campers to provide their own first aid.

Practice Hint
The first bandage is first aid; the second one isn't.

   e. Summoning the nurse at night.

Practice Hint
ALWAYS wear something to bed.

f. Managing common camper health challenges.
- Working with a nauseous camper or one who has thrown up.
- Menarche and menstruation concerns: cramps, having adequate supplies, disposing of used items, "accidents."
- Losing teeth and the camp's Tooth Fairy tradition.
- Monitoring food and water intake; behaviors that indicate an eating problem as opposed to a lack of appetite.
- Strategies to minimize the Cabin Plague (sore throats, common cold): sleeping head-to-toe, washing hands, no sharing, removing wet items from the cabin and onto the clothesline to dry, etc.
- Keeping allergies at bay.
- Coping with "infirmary-itis" (or what to do with campers who think a daily visit to the health center is part of their personal schedule).

g. Describing the growth and development tasks of children; discuss how camp practices complement and/or frustrate those tasks. *Note that this may be covered by someone else; check with the camp director.*

5. Injury management (see "First Aid That Counseling Staff Can Provide"):
   a. Location of first aid kits around camp: what is in them, how the items are used.
   b. Summoning help while maintaining personal safety such as practicing universal precautions.
   c. Providing basic life support: opening an airway (including Heimlich maneuver), doing CPR (location of the camp CPR masks?).
   d. What the nurse will do on the scene.

Practice Hint

Show staff your triage procedure so they (a) can assist per request and (b) can interpret your actions to onlooking campers.

---

e. Discuss management of bystanders and the counselor's role.

f. Describe the circumstances that would trigger the camp's full EMS response and when 911 might be called; discuss who makes these kinds of critical decisions.

6. The health service role during severe weather. Procedures it follows in the event of fire or when a camper is missing.

7. Sanitation when table setting: washing hands before handling table wear, touching nonfood areas of silverware, plates, glasses.

8. What it means for a counselor to develop "Safety Eyes" (maintaining safety awareness during activities and program planning).

9. The philosophy of valuing prevention over treatment.

Orient Staff Who Help in the Health Center

Some camps assign other staff to help in the health center. Sometimes they are part-time helpers: they help on Opening Day, may sit with sick campers, and assist during the nurse's time off. Other helpers may work full time in the health center, which is especially true at large camps. How much orientation a helper needs from the nurse depends on the background of the helper and the helper's job description. Ultimately, the more an assistant knows regarding procedures and health center practices, the better the assistant can function. It is extremely important, however, that the nurse and assistant recognize the difference in their roles. The health center assistant does not make nursing decisions. Rather, the assistant provides reliable observation and accurate reporting of information to the nurse. It is the responsibility of the nurse to interpret findings. The nurse defines the parameters of the helper's ability to act through delegation, a professional skill influenced by the state's Nurse Practice Act.

Talk with the Waterfront Manager

In most camps, it is the responsibility of the waterfront (WF) manager to manage the aquatics program. The nurse should prepare a first aid kit for the WF staff and train them in its use. The WF manager and nurse should agree at what point during a waterfront emergency the nurse will take responsibility for an aquatic victim and how the nurse will be summoned.

Organize the Health Center

The first nurse to arrive at the beginning of the camp season generally sets up the health center. Keep in mind that most health centers are closed over the winter, so it isn't surprising to find the area messy and, perhaps, home to a couple of four-legged visitors like mice, chipmunks, or squirrels. Since the camp's maintenance staff are busy with other tasks, it usually falls to the nurse to clean things up. The camp director knows where to find cleaning supplies! Experienced camp nurses always start with their own room, getting it in shape to function as "home base."

Then it's on to the health center itself. Thoroughly clean the area. Arrange the area to provide space for sick campers, a dispensary for office hours, and an office. Sanitize the bed frames and mattresses (mix 1 Tbsp. bleach in a gallon of water) and locate linen. It's a good idea to put a pillow and blanket on each bed even though overnight patients often use their own bedding (counselors can bring an admitted camper's bedding to the health center).

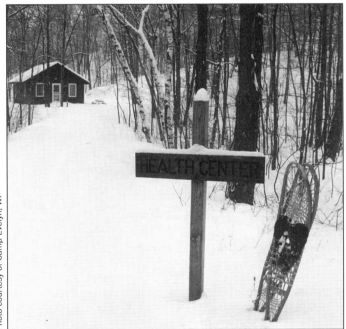

Photo courtesy of Camp Evelyn, WI

31

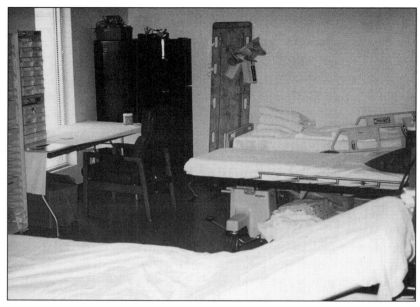

ACA photo file

Locate the nearest phone. Arrange for it to be accessible twenty-four hours a day. Know how to make long-distance calls and how the camp director would like those calls logged.

If the health center doesn't have refrigeration, ice, and hot water, make arrangements for access through the kitchen or another source. Some camp nurses keep a hot pot in the health center and warm water as needed.

Consider security. Medications, including refrigerated prescriptions, those brought by individuals as well as the camp's stock supply, should be locked in a storage area (ACA Standard HW-18).

Practice Hint
Put refrigerated medications in a tackle box and lock the box instead of chaining an entire refrigerator closed!

Determine where health forms and health records will be kept; these too have security implications. Talk with the director about who should have access to these items.

Unpack and organize health center supplies. Ask for a copy of last year's inventory form, and check against it for missing items. Note out-of-date medication and/or inadequate supplies. Report anticipated needs to the camp director (or designated purchasing person).

Practice Hint

Find out if there is a budget for the health center and who has decision-making power regarding that budget.

Also make a locator wheel for the health center door to use when you leave the health center. Most locator wheels are simply a pie chart with a movable hand indicating various places in camp. (In making the locator wheel, consider the wheel's exposure to weather.) The nurse moves the dial to point to the area she or he can be found if needed. Hang the locator wheel and begin using it right away; in other words, start training the staff.

Find out if the camp uses such technological supports as walkie-talkies, pagers, or cell phones to communicate with the nurse on the camp site.

Organize (create?) the record-keeping system (see "Record Keeping").

Meet Local Medical Personnel

Generally, local medical providers will have been contacted by the camp director and agreed to provide services for the camp. Know how to locate the clinic and hospital. Consider preparing written directions to these places (a strategy that may come in handy during an emergency when the person who is supposed to drive just happens to be out of camp). Meet the physician early in the season. Ask about clinic protocol, especially in the business office. Verify clinic hours and phone number. Be familiar with the local hospital's emergency room access and business office procedures.

Locate the dental office. Know its office hours and phone number.

Practice Hint

Find out what time is best for you to call and consult with the camp's physician and/or dentist. Often their nurses can advise you. By getting to know them, you have a "gate keeper" in each office.

Prepare for Emergencies

Post emergency information at all phones. Include written directions to camp and phone numbers for the camp physician, hospital, fire department, sheriff, ambulance, and poison control center.

Identify first aid- and/or CPR-trained staff who could assist you in an emergency. Note which staff are actually *experienced* first aiders.

Explain how to wake the nurse at night and acquaint the counseling staff with this procedure (see "Health Orientation for Camp Staff").

Make first aid kits for the waterfront, kitchen, camp vehicle(s), and other areas — such as the sports field, arts and crafts, cabin areas — as needed. Include simple written instructions. Tape a couple of quarters for emergency phone calls to the inside lid of any first aid kit that leaves the camp (e.g., on vehicles, in trip kits); include the camp's phone and fax numbers. (See Appendix A.)

There are several rules of thumb about first aid kits:

1. Gloves are mandatory.
2. Most kits will simply need adhesive strips, a few gauze pads, a sanitary pad to control big bleeds (not only for menstruation), and some tape.
3. Medications are generally *not* recommended for first aid kits. The health center is usually close enough should a need for medication arise. Too, administration of medication is beyond the scope of first aid training.
4. Consider the geography of camp to determine which kits should contain CPR masks. Obviously, the pool and lake areas need one. The dining room might need one as well.
5. Put a small, spiral-bound notebook and a pen in each kit for staff to document use of the contents. At minimum, require this information:

a. Date and time of incident
b. Legal name of injured/ill person
c. Description of signs and symptoms
d. Description of care provided, including follow-up instructions
e. Signature of person who provided care

> ### Practice Hint
> Use nonlatex gloves everywhere. Most first aid kits get wet at some time during the summer; how waterproof are yours? Check first aid kits during the Walk-around; sometimes the contents walk-away.

The Nurse's Bag

It's important for the nurse to be out and about camp. One needs to see the camp community while it's functioning to more fully understand its needs. Besides, you have to leave the health center to eat, to do the sanitation check (the Walk-around), and to respond to an emergency. To make this mobility possible, fill a backpack or fanny pack with items you need to be functional, and get in the habit of taking this bag whenever leaving the health center.

Known as "the nurse's bag," this vital piece of equipment lets you enjoy camp activities yet also provide care. You can check a skin rash while campers are at the pool or watch a child with a questionable ankle on the athletic field. Inevitably, someone will need something when they see the nurse; carrying the bag helps minimize returns to the health center.

Items typically carried include:

- Small notebook and black pen(s) for record keeping. If you wish, you can carry the health log.
- Indelible black marker (great for marking size of swelling).
- Temperature-taking device. *Note: Choose a device carefully. A mercury thermometer may be a hazard in the bag and devices such as TempaDots are susceptible to high heat. Consider a digital thermometer and use sheaths for infection control.*

- Bandaging supplies (remember a couple of sanitary pads for big bleeds).
- Tweezers for removing slivers/splinters and ticks.
- Medication: carry small amounts of OTCs typically requested when people see the nurse such as acetaminophen, ibuprofen, pseudofed, diphenhydramine, and chlorpheniramine. A word of caution: know the client you are offering the medication to!
- Emergency medication for anaphylaxis (epinephrine).
- Gloves (multiple pairs).
- Instant ice pack.
- Flashlight or penlight.
- Ace wrap (a couple 3" or 4").
- CPR ventilation mask.
- Phone card and phone and fax numbers.

CHAPTER 4

Opening Day: When Campers Arrive

The day that campers arrive is always exciting! Precamp's focus on preparation gives way to implementation. Opening Day is important to the camp nurse too. Medications arrive, screening is done, appropriate staff get updated information about campers with special needs, and the health center begins to officially see clients.

Prepare for Opening Day

At least one day before campers arrive (if not earlier), review health forms in preparation for Opening Day's screening process. The goal of screening is to:

- Update information on health forms, which may have been sent to camp many months earlier.
- Collect both daily and prn medications.
- Verify diet and allergy information.
- Check the health status of incoming people to determine if they pose a risk to the rest of the camp community (communicable disease control).

Practice Hint

Opening Day is the busiest day for most camp nurses. Carefully consider what you want to accomplish and how you'll do it. *Plan this day ahead of time* to minimize harrowing moments.

Many camps have a "screening order" as a part of the camp's protocols. This describes the focus of the camp's screening process and should be used as a guide in designing Opening Day's procedures. (See Appendix B.)

Note: Also screen staff. This is typically done during staff orientation. Talk with the director to determine the appropriate time to do staff screening. Consider using the staff screening to practice Opening Day's procedure so it moves well when campers arrive. See only one staff person at a time. Do not wait until the morning that campers arrive to do staff screening — that makes for a very hectic day! By doing the staff ahead of time, you'll also be collecting their medications and can practice your medication passing process.

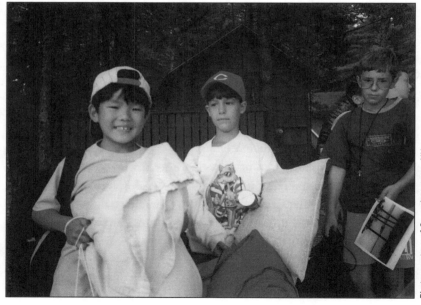

Photo courtesy of Camp Lawrence, NH

■ Assistance May Be Needed for Screening

Unless the camp population is small, it will probably take at least two people to do an effective and time-sensitive screening; sometimes it may take more. Ask the camp director to assign at least one staff member to help on Opening Day and instruct the person about his or her task(s) ahead of time.

■ Prescreen Health Forms

Get an alphabetical or cabin list of incoming campers from the camp office. A suggested pre–Opening Day strategy is to review health forms and, in so doing, code the camper list. Use the coded list on Opening Day to quickly determine needed items from each person as they are screened. An assistant should find using a coded camper list much easier than paging through health forms, and enables you to keep the health forms.

To create a coded list, simply take the first health form and find that person's name on the alphabetical or cabin list. Use the information on that health form to write one or more of the following codes in front of the person's name:

- *Rx* if a medication will arrive with the individual
- *?* if something on the health form needs clarification (e.g., description of an allergic response is incomplete or date for tetanus is lacking)
- *S* if the parent needs to sign the authorization for treatment area
- *OK* if the form is complete, no medication is expected, and nothing needs clarification from a nursing perspective

When all the health forms have been prescreened, the coded list will indicate that some people are uncoded. Those are people from whom you do not have a health form; they will either bring theirs on Opening Day or you will need to complete one with them at the screening.

■ Begin Dietary and Counselor Lists

Camp health forms include information needed by the camp kitchen and tips about an individual that counselors — cabin and/ or activity staff — may need (ACA Standard HW-9). To save time, consider initiating two other forms while prescreening health forms: a diet sheet for the kitchen (see Appendix C) and a notes sheet for counselors.

> **Practice Hint**
>
> Consider the confidentiality of these lists and who will have access to them. A diet list posted in the kitchen may have a different impact than a duplicated copy of camper health needs left inadvertently on someone's clipboard for everyone to read. For this reason, some camp nurses provide only the director with a written record of this information, and simply advise the staff verbally.

Prepare lists for the camp's kitchen staff (head cook) containing this kind of information:

- People with food allergies, specifics about the allergies (e.g., can tolerate milk when used in baked items but not when poured on cereal), and whether the reactions are likely to be anaphylactic or intolerance
- Vegetarians and the type of vegetarian diet followed (e.g., semi, lacto-ovo, pesco, vegan)
- People with special diet needs such as individuals with diabetes, lactose intolerance, or celiac sprue, and notes specific to those needs

> **Practice Hint**
>
> People with diabetes need to know when camp meals are delayed and/or when a change in camp schedule affects the camp's eating pattern.

Give cabin and/or activity staff information affecting a camper's ability to function in the cabin and/or during activities. Examples include:

1. Telling cabin and activity staff about a camper with asthma, what triggers the asthma, and what medication the camper uses to control the asthma. Cabin staff should know where a camper keeps

his or her rescue inhaler(s) at night and make sure the inhaler is with the camper during the day. All staff should know how to help a camper use the inhalers. (See Appendix D.)

2. Explaining characteristics of a camper's seizure disorder, what triggers the seizure, how to prevent or minimize triggers, and what to do if a seizure occurs. Consider the activities this camper will participate in and how to manage seizure activity that occurs during an activity done in the flickering sunlight at the waterfront, or while doing gymnastics, or riding a horse.

3. Informing staff of a child's diabetes management plan, describing the behaviors that indicate he or she may be going into reaction, and what staff should do in the event. (See Appendix E.)

4. Discussing campers with mobility concerns and describing the accommodation plan in place for them.

5. Identifying campers with sleep disorders and providing strategies to minimize, if not eliminate, the impact of the disorders (e.g., keeping them well rested so overtiredness doesn't precipitate sleepwalking and placing known sleepwalkers in bottom bunks).

6. Explaining psychiatric diagnoses that impact cabin life (e.g., AD/HD, Tourette syndrome, Asperger's syndrome, depression) and describing strategies to help the camper in question have a successful camping experience.

7. Identifying campers with sensitivities that need special attention (e.g., anaphylaxis to stings and/or food and increased sunburn potential related to medication).

Practice Hint
If someone has a known anaphylactic reaction, remember to review with staff the procedure for using an EpiPen and how to recognize anaphylaxis.

■ Nurse's List

Some camp nurses also create lists for their own use: noting, for example, campers who keep rescue inhalers so the nurse can monitor use. Other helpful lists include:

- People who have asthma and what triggers a flare for them
- People who respond with anaphylaxis to insect stings/bites
- People who have allergies to medication in the camp's stock supplies
- People who carry personal emergency medications

■ Consider Where and How Screening Is to Be Done

Think about where screening will occur. Some camps have the nurse's screening station at the health center; other camps may set up a table as part of the camp's check-in process. Some camps do aspects of screening — such as head lice checks — as campers board the bus to camp and finish the screening at camp.

No matter where the screening occurs, the location should be sensitive to the need for privacy so people with confidential concerns can speak freely. This sensitivity may exist by virtue of the screening station's physical location (in the health center, for example) or the nurse's sensitivity to a person's needs (e.g., suggesting the person return later for a private conversation). Be aware that some people, when in a public setting, may not indicate their desire for private time; consequently, it is strongly encouraged that the screening station routinely provide privacy.

A growing practice is to have two stations in the screening process. The first station can be handled by a staff member. As it is the first contact campers have with the camp's health services, a friendly, approachable, and up-beat attitude is required (public relations are very important). This station is usually supplied with the coded list of campers, along with pens, extra health forms, pediculosis sticks, and a wastebasket.

The nurse works the second screening station. Medication is collected at this station and privacy should be possible since both verbal and physical exam may occur here. The health center is preferred for this station because everything needed by the nurse is in this area.

Once a screening plan has been thought through, gather the people who will do the screening and talk through the process. The objective is to move campers (and maybe their parents) as quickly as possible but also to provide time to talk with those who need it. In addition, the nurse needs to clarify areas of concern and verify those concerns.

No matter what type of camp, the screening should establish the following minimal requirements for each camper:

- Know how the person is feeling upon arrival.
- Make additions and/or corrections to the person's health form (date and initial these).
- Gather medications — prn and daily — at the health center or, if kept by the individual (e.g, EpiPen or rescue inhalers), a notation is made.
- Be certain the individual poses minimal, if any, threat of communicable disease to others.
- Document each of these items and date and initial them.

Some camps add other components. For example, resident camps at which campers stay four or more weeks often obtain a baseline weight during the screening process. Sometimes campers come for screening in their bathing suits so the nurse can do a visual head-to-toe check. Some camps check temperatures, others look for athlete's foot. Consider what you want to accomplish and then design a system to achieve those goals expeditiously. Screening for communicable disease should take priority but this can be tricky. Checking for head lice, as an example, is often the only *physical* assessment for communicable disease done during the screening process. This check, however, is often accompanied by a question or two about the camper's contact with sick people during the past two or three weeks.

Sample Screening Procedure

This procedure is appropriate for a resident camp of about 130 campers. It uses two people, the nurse and a helper, to accomplish the screening.

Supplies you may need during the screening:

- Health forms for incoming group and blank forms (just in case)
- Coded list of incoming campers
- Several black ink pens, a black indelible marker, a highlighter
- Daily Medication forms

- Pediculosis sticks and a penlight
- Boxes to carry medications
- Labels for attaching information to medication bottles
- Stapler and extra staples
- Nurse's bag — in case your professional skills are needed

The person who works the first station greets the camper, finds his or her name on the coded list, and, at minimum, asks these four questions:

1. How are you feeling now? .... *Expected response: "Fine."*
2. Is there anything that should be added to your health form or has anything changed? ....*Expected response: "No."*
3. Have you brought any medications with you? ....*Expected response: "No."*
4. Have you been exposed to any communicable illness in the last three weeks? ....*Expected response: "No."*

Assuming the answer to each question is as expected and an OK is in front of the person's name on the coded list, the staff member then checks the camper's head for lice (the pediculosis sticks and a wastebasket should be at this table). If the head lice check is negative, the staff member places a check behind the name, and the camper continues on his or her way.

Any deviation in the expected response — meaning that a "yes" answer is given or the head lice check is positive — means that the camper is referred to the second health station after completing all aspects of the first station. A check is still placed behind the referred person's name to indicate that he or she has gone through screening even though the person has an additional step.

All other health concerns are addressed at the second health station by the camp nurse. The health forms are here so the nurse can write additional nursing notes.

- Medications are in-processed.
- Health forms that arrive with campers (those not sent ahead of time) are reviewed.
- New information (changes and/or additions) is added to the form.
- Signs of a health problem are assessed.

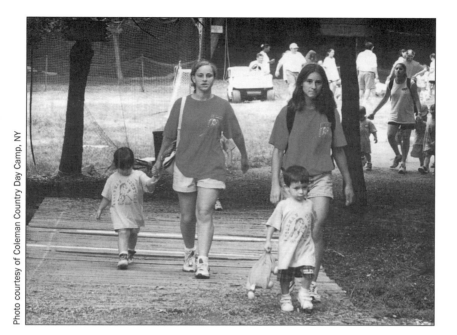

Photo courtesy of Coleman Country Day Camp, NY

- Questionable head-lice checks are verified.
- Written instructions from parents are stapled to the camper's health form.

The second station hosts only one camper at a time to protect privacy concerns. If the station gets too busy, you may want to ask those who are waiting to return when fewer people are waiting. Note the names of people who leave to verify that they do return.

After screening is complete, review all health forms and sign off on a screening note. Verify that each person went through the health screening process. The list becomes part of the health records for that session (file it in the session's folder).

Screening is a critical part of In-processing both staff and campers. It enables the health center to update information, clarify questions, and collect medications. It is also the first line of defense for communicable disease control. Follow a planned screening process and work to completely assess everyone.

45

Opening Day
(*Things to Consider on the Day Campers Arrive*)

Opening day gives the nurse an opportunity to meet the incoming campers and, in some cases, their parents. A stop at the health center is part of the Opening Day process. In addition to functioning as a health screening, this stop also fulfills a public relations function: it's the first time campers and their parents meet the camp's nurse in that professional role. Consider, for example, what you wear and the first impression given by the health center. This might be a time when a white lab coat comes in handy to make it easier to identify the nurse.

Have all screening items ready: health forms, extra (blank) health forms, a large box in which to place medication, a cabin list of who lives where, an indelible marker, self-sticking labels, a couple pens, a pencil, paper, and a stapler.

The objective is to gather adequate information from each person about her or his health. It is just fine — in fact, desirable — to write supporting notes (which should be dated and initialed) on individual health forms as needed, paying particular attention to:

- Describing how an allergic person reacts to the allergen
- Adding parent vacation phone numbers in case of emergency
- Getting the parent signature authorizing treatment for the camper
- Hints about a camper's health idiosyncrasies

With luck, most health forms arrive before the camper's arrival at camp. Some camps, however, allow campers to bring them on Opening Day. Sometimes a camper arrives without a health form. In these situations:

- Have the parent complete a blank health form and sign the authorization statement.
- If the parent is not with the camper, complete as much of the form as possible with the camper's help. This may be done later on Opening Day or the next morning. Note the lack of parental consent and bring this to the camp director's attention. Should the camper require treatment, obtain consent on the phone from the custodial parent followed by written consent. Document this action.

Practice Hint

When a camper doesn't have parental authorization for treatment, consider using nonmedication modalities such as relaxation, massage, and hydration.

All medications are left at the health center on Opening Day. Each medication container must be labeled with the owner's name, name of the medication in the container, dosage, and administration instructions. Use self-sticking labels and/or an indelible marker to provide missing information. *Count daily medications to be certain there is enough to last for the camper's stay.* Consider counting and recording the number of pills for controlled substances (e.g., Ritalin, Cylert).

Giving your medication to a strange person can be extremely anxiety-provoking, especially to campers managing chronic illnesses who are used to controlling their own medications. The nurse can even expect questions from parents should they be present. It is extremely important that everyone understand how to get their medication when needed. Take time to make this clear, especially when a medical condition warrants (e.g., diabetes or asthma), emphasizing where to go for the next dose. Eventually they'll learn the routine!

An exception may be made for rescue (prn) inhalers used to manage asthmatic conditions and/or individual epinephrine delivery devices. There are two ways that camps typically manage this:

1. The camper keeps the device in a fanny pack that is worn all the time except during the night. During sleep, the fanny pack is hung on the camper's bed.
2. The inhaler is carried by the staff member who travels from place to place with that camper's group.

If based on an assessment of a camper's ability to self-manage, you release a medication to be carried by the camper (a) be sure that staff know which camper is carrying what medication and for what purpose and (b) monitor the camper's self-administration.

Some camp nurses write their initials on the inhaler or epinephrine device with an indelible marker. Then staff have a visual cue that this specific medication is appropriate for the camper to carry.

Ask campers to use a fanny pack to carry medications because it's too easy for things to fall out of pockets. It's useful if you have another dose of the medicine for emergency use or in case a device gets lost or damaged. Find out if the camp director asked parents to provide an extra.

One of the most important tasks of Opening Day's screening process is to generate a record of campers' daily medications. Think of a hospital's medication administration record and adapt it to camp. Camps that serve the general population might record the medications of several campers on one Daily Medication Record (DMR), whereas camps with special populations often use one DMR per individual (see Appendix F). Tell the camper where and when to come for the first administration of the medication. Once the first dose is given, it will be easier for him or her to remember routine.

Some state regulations may be restrictive about campers arriving at camp with medications. Some require the medication to arrive in its original package with appropriate labeling in place. Ask about your state regulations and what parents have been told about sending medication with their camper.

Some campers will arrive on Opening Day with prn medications. Check for accurate and legible information on the label: contents, dose, and administration. Label these medications prn and store them apart from the daily medications.

Sometimes parents mix several medications in the same container. Vitamins of various types, analgesics, and cold remedies are classic examples. You may ask parents to identify the pills (confirm that identification using a *PDR*), but *do not administer the medication if any doubt exists as to its identity*.

Some camps give everyone a "camp name." If this is the case, record this name for general use but remember to use the legal name for charting purposes. It may be helpful to record both the legal and camp names on medications.

Remind counselors to double-check for medications that might have slipped into the cabin via camper suitcases. This can be done as campers are unpacking, making their beds, and getting settled in the cabin.

In addition to the medication list, update the kitchen's diet list. At a minimum, update the following:

- Vegetarians/vegan diets
- Food allergies: note which cause anaphylaxis (are truly life-threatening)
- Medically noted diets (e.g., diabetes, lactose intolerance, gluten intolerance)

Ideally, the head cook will have received most of this prior to the first meal. Make special note of foods that are fatal for a given person (e.g., peanut allergies or seafood sensitivity). Be certain that the kitchen staff fully realizes the danger.

Conduct a pediculosis check on all campers and staff within twenty-four hours of their arrival. Document the results of this check and action taken on questionable heads. It is possible for the nurse to train a couple assistants for this task. However, delegation implies that adequate supervision is provided.

Screening is no guarantee that an emerging case of head lice has been caught. Remind counselors to watch for a camper who repeatedly scratches the head and refer him or her to the health center to be checked again.

Complete other areas of physical assessment as needed.

■ Health Talk to Campers

The nurse usually talks to campers early in the session, maybe even Opening Day. This talk informs campers of health and safety issues that affect them. As with the staff orientation, it is important to communicate not only information but also sincerity, competence, and a caring attitude. Presenting a well-planned talk helps convey this message. Introduce yourself and then discuss:

- The location of the health center
- The times of office hours
- How to get help in an emergency — and what constitutes an emergency

- How to get help at night
- What should be done to clean the cabin and when cabin checks are done and by whom
- How to get access to personal prn and daily medications
- Information about the Nurse's Walk-around

CHAPTER 5

In-Session Tasks: Things Done While Campers Are in Camp

Office Hours

One of the camp nurse's primary tasks is to see people with emerging health concerns. This is typically done during office hours (some older camp health models may still use the phrase "sick call" to describe this time). Chapter 6 provides an in-depth discussion of this important topic.

Prevention of Injury and Illness

Injury and illness prevention is a camp priority. Minimizing hazards and managing risk elements is an ongoing concern. A relatively small amount of effort can effectively reduce or eliminate a potential problem and is well worth the invested time. Some areas to note and coach counselors about:

- Are campers dressed appropriately for the weather and/or activity? Campers may need convincing that one can be dressed "in style" yet also in line with what the environment demands.
- Are campers and staff getting adequate rest? If the health center starts to attract fatigue-based problems (e.g., headaches, sore throats, feelings of malaise), talk with the camp director. An earlier bedtime or a modified schedule and/or other strategy may ease the situation.

- Are broken or damaged structures fixed in a timely manner?
- Be aware of and responsive to weather. A series of hot, humid days can quickly establish conditions for heat exhaustion, particularly among staff members. Ask the kitchen to put water pitchers on all tables and speak directly to at-risk personnel (i.e., waterfront, kitchen, and maintenance staff).
- Note the dining room's noise and activity level. This is an excellent barometer of a camp's emotional health. It also affords you an opportunity to approach a listless camper or one who is not eating before he or she becomes too ill and/or emotionally upset.

The Nurse's Walk-Around

The nurse is usually charged with monitoring the camp's cleanliness and sanitation procedures. Overall, camps are usually guided by standard food sanitation procedures and governed by directives from the state health department and the American Camping Association (ACA). Although the procedures for meeting these directives may vary from camp to camp, the underlying principles remain the same. Daily monitoring helps identify a concern before a *bona fide* problem exists. The Walk-around is a public health surveillance procedure; in this situation, the camp is the "public."

Ask the director to explain how the camp meets sanitation standards, adjust those procedures as needed, and tailor monitoring tasks to blend with the overall camp program.

Here are some things to note during the Walk-around:

1. Grounds are free of litter and there's no evidence of septic backup.
2. Windows and doors into sleeping and eating areas are screened and designed to prevent visits by critters of any size.
3. In the cabins:
   a. Floors are moderately clean (the concept of "clean dirt" exists at camp).
   b. Wet and/or damp clothing is hung outside to dry so mold or mildew does not build up in the cabin.
   c. Wastebaskets and garbage containers are emptied daily.
   d. Heads on beds are placed to attain the greatest distance between sleeping people.

e. Toilets are clean and free flowing.

f. Showers are clean and sanitized daily.

g. Hand washing facilities are clean and supplied with soap.

4. Dining tables are sanitized before they are set for a meal.

5. Table setters handle table items with freshly washed hands and in such a manner that eating surfaces are not contaminated.

Check first aid kits during the Walk-around. Restock items and review documentation for appropriate use and/or indications of greater health needs. One idea is to check a different kit each day (kitchen, van, waterfront, crafts, cabins, maintenance), making certain that all are checked at least once in the course of a week. Consider asking the people using the kit if the contents have met their needs.

The food service must comply with strict health regulations. Because the kitchen is usually managed by a head cook, that person should be alerted when the nurse observes poor sanitation techniques in food handling or dishwashing or among personnel. Generally, it is the head cook's responsibility to make sure the food service meets sanitation requirements, not the nurse's.

Special Camp Events

Most camps have special events during the season: Visiting Day, campouts, regatta, Tribal Day, cookouts, Camp Olympics, and so forth. These days, with their special schedules, often affect delivery of medications and treatments. Get in the habit of asking for a schedule as soon as a special day is announced. Consider how to adapt the health center's services and which clients may need special arrangements to support their health needs, and then make those changes.

The camp's *tripping program* is of particular note. Camps take a variety of trips: day trips to historical landmarks, one-night campouts, three- or four-day canoe trips, extended (two weeks or more) trips to remote areas. Healthcare must still be provided when people are away from the main camp site and, thus, remote from the health center and nurse (ACA Standard HW-13).

When trips are announced, get a list of participants — campers and staffers — from the trip leader and review that list to determine

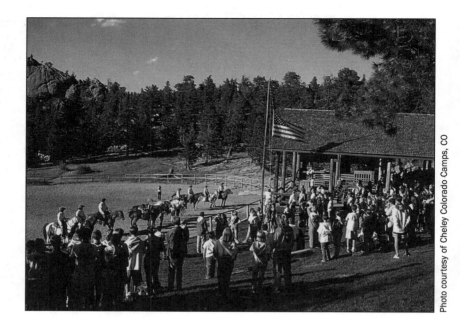

Photo courtesy of Cheley Colorado Camps, CO

the health needs of the individuals. Know the length of the trip, the nature of the trip, and the first aid credential of the staff member assigned to provide healthcare. (See ACA Standard HW-1.) Meet with this person to review what is needed by trip participants. Often this means discussing daily medications, management of individuals with anaphylaxis, and special considerations for certain individuals (who has asthma, who is recovering from a sprained ankle, who is susceptible to heat, etc.). The trip's first aider should carry emergency information specific to each participant.

Pack a trip first aid kit that provides for the needs of the individuals and accounts for the nature of the trip. Note the potential for this kit to include medications. Since on-the-trail decision making with regard to medications is not often a component of the first aider's credential, you may have to teach him or her about the medications being carried. Document this training; from a nursing perspective, such delegation must include a method for monitoring the situation. Some camps, for example, have trips carry a cellular phone so the first aider can call the camp nurse if a health need arises; other camps may hire tripping staff who have had medication management courses.

When planning support for trips, consider the risks to which the group may be exposed. Provide supplies to meet these needs. For example, the risk of anaphylaxis from stinging bees often exists, necessitating the need for epinephrine and diphenhydramine (consider chewable diphenhydramine for trip kits). But also consider how long it may take for someone to be evacuated. When this is factored in, it becomes apparent that a minimum of two doses of epinephrine should probably accompany every trip. Also think about the potential for medications to get wet; consider two medication containers, each in its own dry sack. Having anticipated problems makes a big difference when health concerns surface during trips!

A special category of trips — those lasting three or more nights (sometimes called "tripping programs") — needs one other bit of attention from the camp nurse. ACA Standard PT-9 directs camps to screen camper and staff participants within eighteen hours of departure ". . . to identify any observable evidence of illness, injury or communicable disease that could affect trip participation . . ." (1998; p. 172). Many camps simply have trip participants stop at the health center on the morning of the trip's departure. A better approach would be to do this screening the evening before. Then you have more time to respond to a problem that might otherwise jeopardize someone's anticipated trip.

When Camp Has Multiple Sessions

Many camps have more than one session. For example, eight-week camps may also have campers who stay for four weeks, and then go home on change-over day as another group of four-weekers takes their place. Some camps change camper groups every week while day camps may see population adjustments on a daily basis. This means that you may be working with campers in various programs and/or preparing for the arrival of a new group while completing the stay of the current one.

Practice Hint
Keep paperwork and medications separate, based on session. This makes your life much easier than having everything in a jumble and trying to sort it out on change-over day.

You should prepare for the incoming session during the last few days of the current session. Begin by prescreening health forms. Get a cabin or camper list from the camp office and code it. Note medications that are coming, allergies (particularly those that affect diet) and their antidote, chronic health concerns, and other pertinent information. Make a list of incoming campers with special diet needs and give it to the head cook as soon as possible so she or he can plan menus and order adequate food supplies.

Note which campers have a health concern about which staff should be informed (e.g., bed-wetting, diabetes, sleepwalking, headaches if overtired). Contact the director to learn at what staff meeting you can present this information. Most directors want a briefing on these special needs prior to the staff briefing. Because of confidentiality, remind people to keep written health information in a secure area.

Practice Hint

If questions about a camper arise upon review of the health form, consider calling the parent to discuss the question prior to Opening Day. This saves valuable time for everyone and tells the parents that you are interested in and concerned about their child.

When a session ends:

1. Return medications that were turned in on Opening Day, including empty containers. Some camps do this at breakfast on closing day; the nurse gives the medications to cabin staff who, in turn, put the medications in the campers' suitcases. Other camps, especially those where parents pick up campers, may have parents stop at the health center as part of out-processing.

2. Close out the health records of those who leave. Just as a screening note was made on Opening Day, so too should an exit note be made and unused lines on personal health records "X-ed" out. If the camper is leaving with a current health problem, note the problem and to whom it was referred. All camper referrals *must* be made to a responsible adult (most often the custodial parent). Staff members who are adults can handle their

own referral instructions. Junior counselors and counselors-in-training (CITs), because of their underage status, are usually handled as campers.

Sample Exit Notes

7/14/01 @ 12N: left camp to home. [Signature]
7/14/01 @ 12N: left camp to home. Parents told how to monitor PI recovery. [Signature]

---

3. Move health records for the completed session to the appropriate storage place. Remember to insert additional records such as the Daily Medication Record, copies of insurance forms, diet notes, information given to counseling staff, and notes from external physicians.
4. Check supplies. Order replacement items as needed.

Last Day of a Session

This is another busy day in the health center. Medications are returned and health forms closed. Return containers from empty personal prescription medications in case they are needed for insurance purposes. Be available as much as possible to answer parental questions about camper health.

Some closing programs provide time for the nurse to address the parents. Consider this an opportunity to tell parents what to expect as campers readjust to home life. Talk about the excitement phase on the way home, the desire for "real" food, and the need for rest. Invite parents to contact you if questions about the child's health occur. Perform this task in a professional manner as it may be the only impression the parent receives about the health program. The camp director can offer specific reactions to your closing day comments; ask for that feedback.

Sometimes a camper gets ill the night before going home or is going home looking less than perfect (think of poison ivy on the face, for example). In such an event, it's a good idea to call parents ahead of time. Traveling with a child who is throwing up or has diarrhea should be planned for, and seeing a "perfect child" looking less than perfect because of poison ivy can be a blow to parental expectations.

Health Team Transition

A growing number of camp nurses work only part of the camp season. They transition into camp following another nurse or orient an incoming nurse. Ask the director to schedule an overlapping day so the incoming and outgoing nurses have time to pass critical information along. Think of this as "report." The outgoing nurse can facilitate the transition by doing a tour of camp; introducing key people; providing an orientation to the health center and the camp's emergency system, information about the kitchen, and a report of current individuals' health needs; and describing a routine day for the nurse.

End of Summer

Just as camp was busy before campers arrive, so too do camps have a busy end of season. Ask the camp director about the procedure to close the health center. Often these tasks — like taking inventory — can be started before the final hour. Other areas of attention often include:

1. Nurse's final report: This presents an overall reaction to the job and is designed to assist the camp administration in evaluating the season as well as developing the health services program. The report is usually read by the camp director.
2. Packing supplies for the winter: Specific directions should be given to the nurse. In general, items that can stand freezing temperatures may be stored right in the health center while items that might freeze are sent to a temperature-controlled area for winter storage.
3. Packing records for storage and access by the director during the off-season.

CHAPTER 6

General Practices of a Camp Health Center

Understand the Framework Before Tackling the Specifics

Camp nurses take the responsibility for care of campers and staff very seriously; this is especially true when someone gets ill or injured. Because camps also take this responsibility to heart, the camp often makes promises to parents about how that care will be rendered. Read through the camp's parent information. Note the promises made to the parents with regard to health services and plan delivery of care to complement those promises.

The camp has probably done the same with regard to health services for staff. Read that information too. Remember, however, that there are significant distinctions between caring for staff and caring for campers:

- Campers are clients of the camp, whereas staff are employees. The perception of "How cared for do I feel?" has a different meaning for campers (and their parents) than it does for staff.
- Campers are generally not adults, whereas staff typically are of legal age. Staff can give consent for treatment and make their own decisions; a camper's parents *must* be a part of the decision-making for their child.

59

- As employees, staff are affected by OSHA regulations; campers are not. As employees, staff have access to worker compensation insurance and certain protections (such as OSHA's Bloodborne Pathogen Standard).

Practice Hint

Ask the camp director to explain your role in the camp's OSHA programs. As an employee, you are not responsible for creating these programs; the employer is. You may be asked to help administer the program, however.

You should know if the camp is accredited by the American Camping Association (ACA). ACA-accredited camps follow some basic written policies and procedures specific to health services prepared to comply with the camp's accreditation. Ask for a copy of this material, too.

Also read the *Standards and Scope of Camp Nursing Practice* (Association of Camp Nurses, 2001). These provide a framework for a nursing practice specific to a camp.

With this background, you should focus attention now on the specifics of organizing and managing the health center in order to provide health care that meets the needs of campers and staff.

What follows is a general description of practices common to camp nursing.

■ Office Hours

The health center needs designated times each day — office hours — when it is open to see clients. Office hours should be sensitive to the general camp schedule and long enough to meet client needs. For example, using the half hour of unscheduled time before lunch or dinner is a classic time to be open, whereas opening during cabin duties doesn't work so well (campers quickly learn that claiming to be "sick" gets a trip to the nurse in place of doing their cleanup chores). Some camps have traditional health center hours and others ask the nurse to set the times.

Sometimes a camp nurse will be hesitant to set office hours, preferring "to see people as they need it." While this may be possible in some situations, it also means the nurse is constantly "on," making it tough to plan time for other tasks. Consequently, setting office hours — and sticking to them — is recommended so that people know when you are available for routine matters, and you can provide some structure to your day. At minimum, you should provide time in the morning, afternoon, and evening. Consider using Rest Hour, a time after lunch when people are quiet, for extended treatments like soaking a foot. Have campers bring books to read so they still get the benefit of Rest Hour.

Routine office hours also support the staff expectation that campers will be on time for activities and other planned events. Expect staff to question a camper who reports late to an activity using "The nurse kept me" as an excuse. If this does happen — and it will upon occasion — send a dated and signed note with the camper.

Consider the impact of your office hours on the staff. They often have duties during office hours or may not be comfortable seeing the nurse when campers are present. Because of this, consider providing a "staff-only" time or a special appointments time. Or give staff "priority status" during office hours, and let them go to the head of your line so their concerns can be handled efficiently. Another strategy is to use mealtimes to connect with one another. Use your orientation talk with staff to discuss their access to health services; involve them in making a decision about their need for accessing health services.

Practice Hint

Make it a point, when leaving the health center, to carry your nurse's bag. Then, when staff report the need for something, you can help them right there. It saves time for everyone.

A final comment is important to the topic of office hours. It relates to child protection issues and the sensitivity that today's camps have about protecting children and youth. Office hours at the health center provide opportunity for the nurse to physically assess campers and staff. In doing these assessments, there will be times when you have to examine a private area of a person's body. You should have another adult present — one who is the same gender as the camper. This may be the camper's counselor or another trusted adult of the child's selection. At no time should a camp nurse put his or her own well-intended action in jeopardy by inadvertently doing something that might be misconstrued.

■ Admit Area

The admit area is the place used by campers and staff who spend extended time in the health center. Time may vary from a short nap to an overnight or even longer. Admit space must be gender sensitive. According to ACA Standard HW-15, there should be one admit bed for every fifty people (campers plus staff) in the camp.

Place a pillow and blanket on each bed for short-term use. When considering the use of sheets, first determine the access of a washer and dryer to the health center. If these are convenient, then using more linens is an option. Some camps, however, ask clients who stay overnight to use their own bedding. Counselors can bring the camper's bedclothes to the health center.

Under no circumstances should admitted clients sleep or rest in the nurse's private quarters. Those quarters, which are often only a simple bedroom, should be separate from admit areas but not so far removed that the nurse cannot hear someone at night.

Practice Hint
Use a baby monitor to hear clients during the night. Place the transmitter with the client and the receiver near your bed.

When considering the admit area, also consider how isolation space in case of communicable disease might be provided. This site-dependent decision should make space available which minimizes, if not eliminates, contact with the greater camp community. Isolation is commonly used during the first twenty-four hours that some-one is on antibiotics for strep throat or when a case of chicken pox erupts.

■ Admit Policy

In general, the expectation of a camp is that campers and staff came to participate in the camp's program. Consequently, help a person with a minor injury or illness adjust his or her camp schedule to enable participation. For example, a person with a headache can be given medication but also coached to drink more water and select activities — or adapt an activity schedule — conducive to recovery.

If, however, a person is so ill or injured that she or he cannot participate in camp activity, even with a modified level of activity, that person belongs under the observation of the nurse and should be admitted to the health center. Counselors have their own responsibilities and should not be expected to provide full-time care for an ill or injured camper, nor should they expect such a camper to be sleeping in the cabin.

Be sure to notify the camp office when a camper or staff member is admitted; ask the director what form this communication should take. Camps have designated attendance checks and well-rehearsed "lost camper" drills. It's quite humbling to start that drill only to discover that the lost person is the one recently admitted to the health center! On the other hand, admitting a staff member has implications for activity coverage and so forth. For this reason, some camp directors want immediate notification about staff admits. Just as you inform the camp office of admits, remember to also tell them when a person has been released.

According to ACA Standard HW-16, there must be constant supervision of admitted persons by an appropriately trained member of the staff. Ideally, supervision is provided by the nurse, but consider training other staff to help when duties take you out of the health center (e.g., to pass medications at meals or to do the Walk-around) or when you are off duty or simply on break.

■ Medication and Supplies

Although health center items are usually designated for health use and are only accessible through the nurse, supplies sometimes might serve as props for a play or find their way into a campfire skit! The nurse is responsible for organizing these items so emergency items (splints or epinephrine, for example) can be located easily, and someone other than the nurse can function in the area if an emergency arises. This generally means that:

- Stock medications are grouped by functional need: gastrointestinals are together, analgesics are together, topicals are together, etc.
- Personal medications are stored separate from stock medications and in a way that facilitates quick location (consider alphabetizing them by person's last name).
- Personal medications used daily are separate from personal prn medications.
- Medications are stored in a secured (locked) area. (See ACA Standard HW-18.)
- Emergency medications such as epinephrine are readily available.
- Bandaging supplies are readily available. Note that bandaging supplies are not under a "controlled access" standard; however, consider the client population and make a decision based on the best interests of that group.
- A sharps container and infectious waste receptacle — both with biohazard labels — are in the health center.

Camp nurses often wonder what should be stocked in a health center. When determining the items for a specific health center, consider:

- Profile of the campers and staff — are they generally in good health or do they have special needs?
- Profile of the camp's activities — are there particular injuries that you should be prepared to handle?
- Profile of illnesses — if people are at camp more than one week, the potential for illness increases. Be prepared for URI and GI processes.

64

Suggested Health Center Supplies

■ Bandaging Supplies

Adhesive strips
Benzoin
Conforming gauze rolls
Elastic wraps, 3" and 4"
Gauze pads, sterile
Gauze sponges, nonsterile

Knuckle bandages
Large bandages
Steri-Strips
Suture removal kit
Tape, 1" and ½"

■ General Supplies

Alcohol preps
Allergy syringes, 1 cc
BP cuff (child and adult sizes)
Cold packs, instant
Cotton-tipped swabs, 3"
CPR barrier mask
Crutches (various sizes)
Eye shield
Eye wash
Eyeglass repair kit
Gloves, disposable (nonlatex)
Isopropyl alcohol
Liquid soap in pump dispenser
Masks
Medication cups

Medication envelopes
Orthodontic supply kit
Peak flow meter
Pediculosis sticks
Penlight
Provo-iodine soak solution
Sanitary pads and tampons
Scissors
Splinter forceps
Stethoscope
Thermometer device and shields
Tongue depressors
Toothbrushes
Vomit clean-up chemical

■ Medications (with abbreviations)

Acetaminophen (APAP), 325 mg
Acetaminophen chew tabs
Aspirin (ASA), 5 gr
Baking soda
Bismuth (note: salicylate)
Calamine lotion
Chlorpheniramine maleate, 4 mg
Diphenhydramine, 25 mg
Epinephrine 1:1000 (epi)
Guaifenesin D (dextromethorphan)
Head lice treatment
Hydrocortisone cream, ½% and 1%

Ibuprofen, 200 mg
Ipecac syrup
Kaolin-Pectin
Mediplast
Poison ivy treatment
Pseudoephedrine, 30 mg
Salt (for saline gargles)
Silver sulfadiazine
Throat lozenges
Tolnaftate
Triple antibiotic ointment (TAO)
Vinegar

■ Office Supplies

Black, indelible markers
Black pens
Boxes to build first aid kits
Clipboard
Disposable camera
Documentation supplies
Health forms (blank)
Highlighter

Ice
Labels, self-adhesive
Nurse's drug reference and other
    references as needed
Refrigerator lock box
Safety pins
Baggies and/or paper bags

- Last year's inventory — compare what remains with what was ordered. You can quickly see what items must be replaced or are in high demand as well as items that rarely or never get used.
- Physician's treatment protocols — since your ability to administer medication is governed by the camp physician's treatment protocols, stock only those medications specifically mentioned in the protocol by the physician.

Keep an eye on supplies. The quantity needed at the start of summer is different from that needed by the end of the season. Also note Appendix G.

■ Sanitation

To maintain a clean and sanitary health center, sweep floors daily, empty wastebaskets routinely, maintain admit beds with "throw up buckets" tucked within reach, and sanitize toilet facilities and treatment areas daily. Assess the health center's air flow; if needed, augment air flow by strategically placing fans. Keep disposable cups, towels, and tissues on hand — as well as a large wastebasket.

Some camps provide housekeeping services to the health center; others expect the nurse to clean as needed.

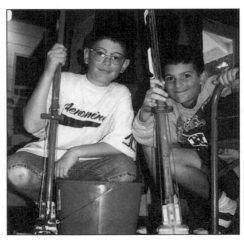

Photo courtesy of Menominee for Boys, WI

Sanitizing Solution

Using a 1-quart spray bottle, mix 1 quart of water with $1/8$ teaspoon common bleach. This simple sanitizing solution, which results in a solution of 50 parts per million, can be used to wipe down health center surfaces and sprayed on surfaces and allowed to air dry.

Note that chlorine breaks down over time, exposure to air, and exposure to proteins. Consequently, either mix a new solution daily or — better yet — use the sanitation test strips from the kitchen. These look like pH litmus test strips.

■ Leaving the Health Center

It is acceptable — and encouraged — for the nurse to leave the health center and generally be available within the camp. Some camps provide the nurse with a pager, walkie-talkie, or cellular phone for these times; others may have the nurse simply tell the office where to find him or her if needed. The bottom line is that campers and staff quickly learn to head over to the health center when there's a problem, whether it be a minor thing or a huge emergency. Consequently, when a camp nurse leaves the health center, it is recommended that the following be done:

1. Secure the health center from curious campers and staff (e.g., medication cabinets are locked and health records are closed).
2. Post a message on the door telling when the nurse will return, where she or he can be found, and where to find help in case of emergency.
3. Arrange for admitted clients to be supervised by a staff member trained for the task.

■ Identifying an "Epidemic"

Typically, as the camp season wears on, you will see so many people with common human problems — upset stomachs, headache, sore throat, abdominal cramps — that it's quite possible to overlook an emerging epidemic. Consider this rule of thumb: *when any three or four people report to the health center with the same symptoms within a three-hour period, consider what else might be happening.*

Epidemics are not common in camps; in fact, they're fairly rare. But they certainly are a possibility. Food-borne illness and Norwalk virus are typical culprits. When you suddenly find the admit beds full and three more people vomiting on the front steps, the time to recognize a need for assistance is long gone. Keep an eye on the flow of client complaints and plan for the eventuality of an epidemic ahead of time. Talk with the camp director about:

- Defining an "epidemic" for camp: at what point does the director want to be notified of a potential problem?
- Creating more bed space: can a cabin become a ward?
- Getting more nursing support: are there local nurses who can be on call?
- Responding to the increased demand on supplies: more linens, additional laundry runs, additional emesis basins (ice cream buckets work great!), more clear fluids, etc.
- Contacting out-of-camp people — when and who calls them: state Department of Health, local physician, camper parents, insurance carrier, media.
- Changing camp practices to break the chain of communicability: eat meals outside, keep "near sick" away from those with definitive symptoms as well as the nonsymptomatic population, require activities that keep people at least an arm's distance apart from one another, rigorously monitor hand washing, etc.

■ Using a Camera in the Health Center

This item is becoming a more common piece of equipment for health centers but before using a camera, know about the camp's photography release for campers. Also recognize that photos taken in the context of the nurse's job are the property of the camp; such photos should not be used for other purposes.

Consider photographing injuries of suspicious origin or using the camera to document progress of a condition (e.g., rash, wound, burn, etc.). Keep a record of photos by creating a camera log and documenting:

1. Photo number
2. Legal name of subject of photograph
3. Date, time, and place of photo
4. Name of person taking the photo
5. Reason for photograph (what were you trying to capture?)
6. Other information as needed

> **Practice Hint**
>
> Consider the value of digital images. For example, one camp nurse snapped a photo of a wound over which a question about need for stitches was raised. She sent the photo to the consulting physician along with her plan of care. The MD supported the plan based on the photo, and time and money for a clinic run were saved.

■ Regarding Stitches

In this era of skin-closing adhesives and adhering steri-strips with benzoin, at some point, you will probably consider if a given wound should be seen by a physician or if you might close it. If you think stitches may be needed or wonder about a wound's healing prognosis, consult the camp physician and the camper's parents. Some physicians are adamant about stitches, especially for active kids at camp, preferring them to steri-strips or adhesives. And most parents feel that they have a vested interest in the decision. It is not your prerogative to decide for either party. Explain the options and let the parents along with the physician decide. This discussion should take place so the camper is not alarmed.

Staff, as adults, make this decision for themselves.

■ Admission to a Hospital

While certainly feasible, the need to hospitalize campers and staff is generally low. The camp's risk-reduction initiatives make this potential fairly low — but it can still happen. Consult with the camp director about the camp's hospitalization policy. Notification of parents/guardian, coordination of follow-up care, and custodial questions pertinent to campers must all be considered.

■ When a Camper Goes Home Sick or Injured

Sometimes a camper may get so ill or badly injured that the question of having her or him go home is raised. In general, this decision is made in consultation with the camper's parents, the camp director, and a physician. Note that you should not make a decision to send a camper home without consulting the camp director because there are concerns such as coordinating with parents and the camp's refund policy to consider.

In these situations, the nurse often functions as a case manager. Keeping everyone informed is a priority. Use the following guidelines in making a decision:

1. Know the camp's policy about sending campers home. Know it with regard to staff as well, although concerns about an employee are different from those of a camper.
2. If a communicable disease such as chicken pox is involved, recommend that the person go home. Infectious diseases are a serious concern for immunocompromised people.
3. If a camper is admitted to the health center longer than twenty-four hours, the possibility of going home should be discussed with the director and the parents. Sometimes this situation requires contingency planning (e.g., if no improvement in the next twelve hours, then the parents will come for the camper).
4. If recovery would be enhanced by being at home, the question of going home should be raised.
5. If a chronic condition (e.g., asthma) flares to the point that it causes a camper to spend more time in the health center than in the program, going home should be discussed.

Sometimes campers leave camp at the end of their session with a health concern (e.g., slight injury, poison ivy, common cold). Because of this compromised state, call the parents and talk with them about the situation to prepare them for what they might see and to discuss postcamp care. Record this process on the person's health record. Preparing parents is particularly important when a camper has the flu and/or diarrhea because travel plans may need adjustment. Always advocate in the best interest of the camper.

■ Supervising Unlicensed Assisting Personnel

Some health centers are so busy that the camp hires assistants to help the nurse. Determine what credential these people hold and assign their tasks within the parameters of that credential.

It is your responsibility to monitor the assistants' performance. In general, healthcare assistants may gather information about clients, but they report that information to the supervising RN who then makes decisions based on the information.

Tasks typically delegated to assisting personnel include (a) helping with Opening Day's screening process, (b) monitoring admitted clients, (c) assisting with medication administration but not directing it, (d) making beds and cleaning the health center.

Those people who are student nurses or graduate nurses in other settings may *not* be called "nurse" during their camp employment. The title "nurse" is a legally protected title. It may only be used by individuals licensed by the state to practice nursing.

■ Camp Parents: Consider Their Needs Too

Most camps consider their relationship with camper parents/guardians to be quite precious. After all, they decided that their most important focus — their children — will attend a certain camp. During the process of selection, a growing number of parents are asking about the camp's health services. As a result, camp directors will have made certain agreements with parents that impact the camp nurse's role, the way tasks are accomplished, and the scope of care provided by the camp.

Look at the camp's parent materials. Note the comments about health care, and plan care delivery to meet those expectations.

Pay particular attention to comments about communication with parents. According to ACA Standard HW-17, the camp should have implemented a policy specific to parent/guardian notification "that identifies the situations when parents will be notified of an illness or injury to their camper" (American Camping Association, 1998; p. 65). Follow the camp's policy.

In general, camps recognize that parents/guardians have a right to know about and be involved with the health concerns of their child.

When a child is sick or injured, have a plan in mind for caring for the child which can be presented and discussed with the parent/guardian during a call. In addition to providing substance to the phone conversation, it also demonstrates competence. Avoid statements such as "Your child says his ear hurts; what do you want me to do?" A parent who hears that from a nurse has little option but to say, "Take him to the doctor."

Some camps bill parents/guardians for out-of-camp services received by their camper; in such a situation, it's even more important that parents/guardian be kept informed and consulted in the decision-making process.

In an Emergency

Know the camp's parent notification policy and follow it. It's understandable that you or the camp director would establish immediate contact by phone in an emergency (emergency phone numbers and a request to contact are usually recorded on individual health forms). Document these contact points, including attempts to contact the parent/guardian, in the client's health record and summarize the information relayed.

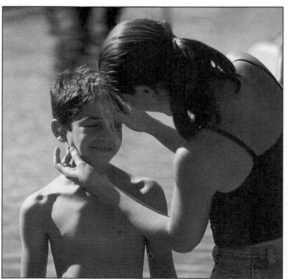

Photo courtesy of Aire Stenberg, CA

When It's Not an Emergency

If, in your opinion, a camper needs referral to an out-of-camp provider (e.g., a physician or an orthodontist) for routine healthcare, you will generally want to talk with the parent/guardian before the child is seen. This important conversation can be used to anticipate outcomes as well as confirm the parent or guardian's availability for consultation should need arise. A follow-up call is often made after the out-of-camp provider has been consulted. In some situations, the camper also talks with the parent/guardian. In addition, talk with the parents/guardians when the camper's recovery pattern deviates from the expected course (e.g., the child doesn't respond to an antibiotic).

A growing number of camps are providing parents/guardians with written documentation of out-of-camp referrals. A letter is often sent within twenty-four hours of the referral and a copy filed with the individual's health record. These letters often include:

- The nature of the illness/injury
- The date of the physician's examination
- The physician's name, address, and phone number
- The doctor's diagnosis and prognosis
- A description of what was done as follow-up at the camp
- Recommendations for follow-up care at home
- The name, phone number, and address of the person who can respond to follow-up questions
- Other information necessary for the incident

■ Physicians: Their Role in Camp Health

Physicians have a variety of roles in organized camping. Some camps have physicians who live on site and see clients much like they would at a home clinic. Other camps may have a physician on the camp Board whose role is limited to providing medical guidelines for the camp. Other camps affiliate with a local physician who agrees to see campers and staff with emerging medical concerns.

From a camp nurse's perspective, a physician's ability to prescribe, diagnose, and order labs and x-rays is a necessary complement to the nurse's skills. Physicians treat injury and illness; nurses treat individuals' reactions to injury, illness, and life events. The two professional roles are complementary.

Consequently, a camp nurse will work with at least one physician who, at minimum, signs the treatment protocols that enable the nurse to provide medication services at camp. In this limited relationship, it is important for the nurse to understand the scope of the protocols in order to avoid overstepping practice boundaries.

Some camps have a long-standing relationship with a physician who has helped the camp develop health and safety procedures tailored specifically to meet the needs of that camp program. This physician often signs the treatment protocols but may also oversee the purchase of health center medications, review the camp's health policies, and serve as an adviser for the nurse.

In addition, camps often access a local clinic and hospital for needed medical services. The doctors in these settings may not be familiar with the organizational framework of the camp. Consequently, the nurse may need to act as a case manager and help the physician understand the level of care the camp can provide.

Make a point of visiting the camp's designated clinic, hospital, and dentist before their services are needed. Ask about in-house preferences for patient care, determine if the office nurse is available for consultation, and check business office procedures. Be sensitive to the doctor's needs also. Areas for consideration include

- Knowing whom to call for an appointment
- Alerting the physician to a special-needs camper before his or her arrival at camp
- Having paperwork accurately completed before arriving for a clinic appointment
- Providing an accurate and complete client history
- Attending to ordered follow-up care in a professional manner
- Sending a responsible adult who is familiar with the case to accompany minors during clinic appointments
- Keeping parents informed and/or arranging for them to talk with the physician

Accompanying a Camper to a Clinic

Campers under legal age are usually accompanied by a responsible adult when receiving medical services from out-of camp providers. This may be the nurse but you could train another staff person to assist with routine physician office visits. Whatever the case, the accompanying adult should be present during examination and/or treatment and gather accurate information about follow-up care. Be sensitive to gender in these situations.

Paperwork

When a client sees an out-of-camp provider, the individual's health form (or a copy of it) is typically sent along or faxed. This paperwork includes parental permission for treatment and should be returned to camp.

Preparing a Camper to See the Physician/Dentist

Receiving medical attention is a stressful event for some people. It can be all the more stressful when away from home, when seeing an unfamiliar doctor, or when feeling a lack of control over what is going to happen. Because of this, take time to honestly prepare the child for what will happen during the appointment. It is also reassuring for the camper to know that someone she or he knows will go along. Most clinics and hospitals used by camps know that the children are away from their usual support systems and, as a result, make a special effort to be sensitive to the child. Camp nurses can facilitate this by having the camper wear something that identifies the child as a camper; camp T-shirts are great for this!

Impact on Camp

Someone leaving camp for a doctor appointment can be disruptive: meals may be delayed, other tasks interrupted, and activities missed. It is difficult to avoid these inconveniences but they should be minimized as much as possible by scheduling appointments at the most opportune time.

If a staff member must see the physician, consult the camp director early so adequate task coverage can be arranged. Staff who are ill or injured impact cabin groups, activity schedules, and a host of other camp functions.

■ Camp Food Service and Health

Many camps take pride in their food service. Meals are nutritious and quality is highly valued. Some camps serve family style so everyone eats a common menu; other camps use a cafeteria model and offer an expanded selection of food. No matter what the situation, the camp's head cook is responsible for the sanitation concerns of the food service program. Camp nurses often support the cook in this area. For example, the nurse might reinforce the need for table setters to wash their hands before doing table duties.

There are a host of food sanitation concerns — largely beyond the scope of this book — but these concerns are taken quite seriously at most camps. This involves who has access to the kitchen, what happens to food that is returned to the kitchen after a meal, and how ill kitchen workers are treated.

At most day camps, campers bring their own lunch. In these settings, make certain adequate water is available, that lunches are appropriately stored, and that campers do not share (or swap) food.

At resident camps, the nurse interfaces with the camp kitchen in several ways. Consequently, get to know the head cook early in the camp season. This allows you both to organize effective procedures rather than react to the stress of a given moment. For example, the health center often needs access to supplies such as ice, juice, fresh fruit, salt, baking soda, vinegar, and "sick camper" food. With the head cook, determine the most convenient time to get sick trays for admitted clients, what items will be available for upset stomachs, and who is responsible for putting the sick tray together.

Anaphylactic reactions to food are a genuine concern at camp. Use the health forms to generate a written list for the kitchen staff of who is allergic to what foods. Make a distinction between food intolerance and anaphylactic responses. Writing these lists helps avoid confusion and forgetfulness (see Appendix C). Make arrangements as

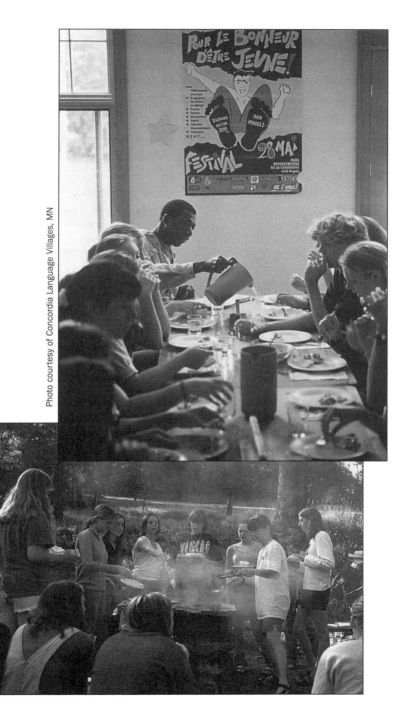

Photo courtesy of Concordia Language Villages, MN

Photo courtesy of Cheley Colorado Camps, CO

77

needed to manage food allergies. In particular, review the menu to determine when foods containing the allergen in question will be served and arrange with the head cook for an alternative. It is a good idea to highlight the food in question so the kitchen staff can alert you if a change occurs.

Anaphylaxis to foods:
A life-threatening situation!

1. Make sure the kitchen staff understands who will react with anaphylaxis and to what food(s).
2. Review the kitchen menu for the item and highlight that dish.
3. DO NOT serve food to which someone may react with anaphylaxis until the individual has been notified.
4. Remember to consider candy in the camp store. There are plenty of hidden nuts in some of that chocolate!
5. Caution cabin staff about "care packages," which may contain items in which the food item is hidden.

While not life-threatening, a food intolerance can make a person quite miserable. Consider interviewing the intolerant individual to determine his or her ability to self-manage and adapt nursing interventions to complement that ability.

A growing number of camps offer a vegetarian alternative menu. Some camp kitchens are fairly adept at working with vegetarian diets while others are less knowledgeable. You may be the person responsible for collecting information about vegetarians.

Pay attention to the diet information on the camp health forms. Parents have signed off on this form. If a deviation is suspected, call the parent to verify the change/adaptation and chart that information on the person's health form. Most camps do not allow a camper to "suddenly convert" to a vegetarian diet since (a) parents have an expectation of a regular diet and (b) kitchen orders for food supplies may not support a change in quantity. Staff who want to try a vegetarian plan are legal adults and may make this decision for themselves. But even they should talk with the head cook before switching since the cook's food orders and staff work loads are affected. It is ultimately the head cook who gives an "OK" for staff to switch to the vegetarian plan.

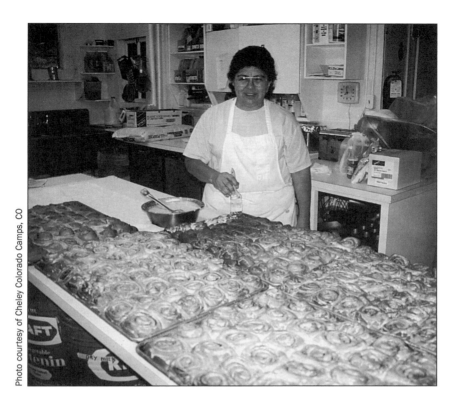

Photo courtesy of Cheley Colorado Camps, CO

Note that in many camps only qualified personnel have access to the kitchen. The food service follows stringent state health regulations that vary significantly from most homes, and the typical counselor does not know these procedures. In addition, the more people who have access to food sources, the greater is the opportunity for contamination of the entire camp population. Consult with the head cook when questions arise about food safety.

Talk with the head cook, and then the whole kitchen staff, about reporting their own illnesses and treating minor injuries using the kitchen first aid kit. Document this training. Kitchen personnel should not work if they have diarrhea; a cold; a running sore, boil, or infected finger/hand; dysentery, TB, or a positive test for typhoid. They must wash their hands after going to the toilet, using a handkerchief, handling dirty utensils, handling garbage, and smoking. Teach them effective hand-washing techniques.

Considerations
Regarding Individuals and Food

If a person is lactose intolerant:

- Can the person tolerate milk products in baked goods?
- Does the person self-manage intolerance by using a product like Lactaid? If so, he or she may not need a special-diet meal from the camp kitchen.
- Can the camp kitchen provide a lactose-free milk substitute?
- Is the person capable of carrying a pocket-pack of Lactaid for use at other than mealtimes?

If a person has diabetes:

- Does the person need access to snacks from the kitchen? If so, at what time(s) and what is needed for a snack (protein, carbohydrate)?
- Introduce this person to the kitchen staff; they should know the individual by sight so they're prepared to get a food item immediately if the individual is unable to ask. Hint: simply pour a glass of milk or juice and coach the person with diabetes to drink it.
- Delayed meals impact people with diabetes! Arrange "Plan B" if a camp meal is delayed. Remember to consider days when mealtimes may change.

If a person is vegetarian:

Find out what kind of vegetarian diet is followed.
- Semivegetarians do not eat pork or beef.
- Pesco vegetarians do not eat pork, beef, or chicken.
- Lacto-ovo vegetarians do not eat pork, beef, chicken, fish, or seafood.
- Vegans do not eat pork, beef, chicken, fish, seafood, dairy, or eggs.

If a person has an egg allergy:

- Are eggs tolerable when used as an ingredient, such as eggs in cookies, cakes, and sauces?

If a person has a peanut allergy:

- Determine the level of sensitivity. Some individuals actually have to eat the peanut before their reaction is triggered, while others may even react to aerosolized particles (someone cracking open peanuts in the shell, for instance).

CHAPTER 7

Record Keeping

*Just as in any clinical setting,
the camp nurse is responsible for maintaining
accurate and complete health records. These are
legal documents; consequently, procedures regarding format, content, and disposition
of information are important.*

Individual Health Forms

Each person — staff and camper — should have a health form on file in the health center. The individual health form is the heart of the health record system. According to ACA Standards HW-2 and HW-6, the health form should contain both history (completed within six months of program participation) and, for resident campers and staff, a medical evaluation (done within two years of program participation). Most camp nurses find it easiest to alphabetize the forms and store them in an area that is accessible but that can be secured, as well.

Note that parent authorization to treat their camper, a minor, is on the health form. Occasionally, this authorization may not be signed. Talk with the camp director about handling this situation. At many camps, the nurse contacts the parent by phone for a verbal authorization *if the child needs treatment*. Document this permission-by-phone on the health form by noting date, number called, person spoken to,

For Office Use

Year

Health History and Examination Form for Children, Youth and Adults Attending Camps   FM 08N

Suggested for resident camp use.

Developed and approved by
American Camping Association
American Academy of Pediatrics

Dates of Camp Attendance _____

Mail this form to the address below by _____ (date)

The information on this form is not part of the camper or staff acceptance process, but is gathered to assist us in identifying appropriate care. Health history (first three pages) must be filled out by parents/guardians of minors or by adults themselves. Update required annually. Health exam (back page) must be completed by approved licensed medical personnel at least every two years.

Cabin or Group

Name _____ _____ _____   Birth date _____ Age at camp _____
        Last   First   Middle

Home address _____
             Street address   City   State   Zip

Social security number of participant _____   Gender: ☐ Male   ☐ Female

Custodial parent/guardian _____   Phone _____

Home address _____
(if different from above) Street address   City   State   Zip

Business address _____ City _____ State _____ Zip   Phone _____

Second parent or guardian or emergency contact _____

Address _____   Phone _____
        Street address   City   State   Zip

Business address _____   Phone _____

If not available in an emergency, notify:

Name _____

Relationship _____   Phone _____

Address _____
        Street address   City   State   Zip

Insurance Information

Is the participant covered by family medical/hospital insurance?   ☐ Yes   ☐ No

If so, indicate carrier or plan name _____ Group # _____

▶ Photocopy of front and back of health insurance card must be attached to this form.

Important — These boxes must be complete for attendance*

Parent/Guardian Authorizations: This health history is correct and complete as far as I know. The person herein described has permission to engage in all camp activities except as noted.

I hereby give permission to the camp to provide routine health care, administer prescribed medications, and seek emergency medical treatment, ordering x-rays or routine tests. I agree to the release of any records necessary for insurance purposes. I give permission to the camp to arrange necessary related transportation for me/my child.

In the event I cannot be reached in an emergency, I hereby give permission to the physician selected by the camp to secure and administer treatment, including hospitalization, for the person named above. This completed form may be photocopied for trips out of camp.

Signature of parent/guardian or adult camper/staffer _____

Printed Name _____   Date _____

I also understand and agree to abide by any restrictions placed on my participation in camp activities.

Signature of minor or adult camper/staffer _____   Date _____

Name

*If for religious reasons you cannot sign this, contact the camp for a legal waiver which must be signed for attendance.

Copyright 1983 by American Camping Association, Inc.   Revised 1990, 1992, 1994, 1995, 1996, 1998, 1999, 2000.

American Camping Association Health History and Examination Form
for Children, Youth and Adults Attending Camps — FM 08N

82

and content of the conversation. Request that the parent send a written authorization statement as soon as possible; in fact, consider the possibility of a faxed statement. Remember to document unsuccessful attempts to contact designated persons; this may be crucial information in some cases.

Some parents may alter the wording of the health form's authorization statement to more accurately reflect the parent's desire for healthcare. In general, follow what a parent directs but also tell the director about the requested variation.

Parents may also provide additional health information (e.g., a letter from their MD, allergy information, medication or treatment orders). Insert this information into the individual's health form; note the date it was received. If the information will be returned to the person when he or she leaves the camp (e.g., allergy desensitizing regimes), photocopy the material so a record remains with the camp file.

Note that staff health information, because of OHSA regulations, should be separate from that of campers.

Documentation

In addition to the health form, you need a system to document nursing notes which should reflect nursing process. As people come to the health center for care, record the date and time, reason for their visit, assessment information, treatment plan, and evaluation criteria. Sign the nursing note. (See ACA Standard HW-19.)

Options available to record nursing notes include:

- ACA's *Camp Health Log*: This is a low-cost, spiral-bound book with numbered pages. Each page can be dated and data entered in columns: time, name, reason for visit, treatment, initials. The system has very limited space for nursing notes; it was designed for use by first aiders but can be adapted for your use.
- Commercial computer-based systems: These programs are costly in comparison to paper-and-pen systems and require a person to input data from the health form into the computer system. To date, the only program designed specifically for a camp health center is *MediPal*. This program has four levels of security and

enables the printing of documented information. An administrative archival function helps protect against unauthorized changes.

- Self-designed computer systems: Developed by individuals, these often make use of a data base to provide notation and/or medication documentation. Security of these systems is questionable and must be addressed if they are to be used for health center documentation.
- Self-designed pen-and-paper systems: Ideas for these range from bound notebooks with numbered pages (available through office supply businesses) to individual nursing notes similar to those used in hospital settings. If you are developing this type of system, write a policy statement that describes procedure and is sensitive to the following:

1. *Write legibly!* There is *no* excuse for being unable to read a written record.
2. Use black ink to record entries.
3. Use legal names when documenting healthcare.
4. Date and record the time of each entry.
5. Each entry must be initialed by the person providing the care. Establish a place to record signatures, initials, and credentials.
6. Chart all care, consultations, phone contacts, and/or medications.
7. Document the reason for accessing healthcare (subjective), observations and/or symptoms noted (objective), a description of the provided care, the rationale for that care, and the results (evaluation) of the care. Documentation must reflect the nursing process.
8. Note changes that deviate from expected recovery patterns.
9. Close each person's record at the end of his or her stay. Note unresolved concerns and to whom the referral for care was routed. Include information about instructions provided.
10. Draw a line through unused space. "X" out unused charting space. Do not skip lines or leave lines unfilled.

All nursing action for individuals should be documented, including out-of-camp referrals (to dentists, doctors, etc.) and medication given on a daily basis. Administration of medications can certainly be part of the routine record system, but you might also create a Daily Medication Record to expedite such charting (Appendix F; see also "Medication Management").

Record keeping should also include notes specific to Opening Day's screening process. At a minimum, record:

1. The person's state of health upon arrival
2. Medications the person gave to the health center
3. Changes made on the health form
4. The individual's exposure to communicable disease within the past three weeks
5. The results of the person's head lice check

Confidentiality

Health forms and the information they contain are confidential. At no time should health records be left unattended in a location other than the health center. In addition, take care that records open on your desk are not accessible to the inquisitive eyes of others (campers or staff). Access should be limited to people you and the camp director specify.

Some staff need information about certain situations and individuals. For example:

1. Activity areas such as aquatic, ropes course, and equestrian should know who has a history of seizure disorders.
2. Food service staff should be told who is allergic to what foods and the extent of the reaction (intolerance or anaphylaxis).
3. Cabin staff need to know:
    a. About campers who take medication for which the therapeutic effect should be monitored (e.g., effectiveness of Ritalin, adverse reaction to an antibiotic)
    b. Who has a history of sleepwalking
    c. Who may experience a severe fear reaction to a given situation (severe storms, spiders, etc.)
    d. Who has a medical condition that may impact cabin life (e.g., Tourette syndrome, Asperger's syndrome)

Worker Compensation

Staff members injured or growing ill as a result of the job are entitled to file for worker compensation insurance. This insurance is mandated and monitored by the state in which the camp is located. Camp staff should immediately contact their supervisor if they are injured or become ill as a direct result of their job, but sometimes they are first seen in the health center. If you believe the incident falls under the auspices of Worker Compensation, contact the camp director, who has specific paperwork to file.

CHAPTER 8

Medication Management

*What am I supposed to do with medications?
Can a counselor help pass meds? What do I do with
meds when trips go out? Can I make up my own
charting record? Do all medications really have to be
kept in the health center?*

These are just a few of the questions surrounding the management of medication in the camp setting. Understanding the nuances of the responses provides the framework that the camp nurse uses to make effective and informed medication management decisions.

Context of Medication Management at Camp

Many campers and staff, in their at-home world, monitor their own health status. Self-care is taught and reinforced by primary care physicians and nurses. As a result, when people come to camp, they often come with the expectation that they will continue to manage their own medication. Yet the camp, acting *in loco parentis*, has its own way of delivering healthcare. One of the distinctions is that medication — all medication — is kept in the health center. "Surrendering" one's medication may feel quite alienating to some.

Frustration may also be felt by the camp nurse. In most settings you work to help clients understand their medications and assume responsibility for self-administration. Yet as camp nurse, you function as part of "The Camp," the group acting *in loco parentis*. Because of this, you must follow camp practices. These practices state that medications are "collected" and "in the controlled possession" of specific people who have responsibility for dispensing meds (see ACA Standard HW-18). Camps have a vested interest in knowing who is taking what medication, for what reason, at what time, and if the therapeutic effect is appropriate. Camps are held to a standard of practice expected of those in the business of caring for children.

Factor in the premise that medication is being used more extensively than ever before. Some substances, such as vitamins, are routinely taken for prevention. Other medication and patient-education practices now enable people with disorders once hard to manage to participate in camp: children with diabetes determine their own insulin needs, and lactose-intolerant individuals use products such as Lactaid. In addition, people are using medications prescribed by different doctors with different specialties; consequently, the potential for drug interaction has grown.

In these circumstances, camp nurses, recognizing that their job includes responsibility for medications, need to know about the camp's routine practices before trying to organize a medication management program. This is especially important if they are asked to delegate medication administration to other camp staff (e.g., trip staff or the person who covers on the nurse's day off).

Lishner and Busch (1994) did the only study that examined delivery of medication to children in summer camps. This research, which used a nonrandomized convenience sample, looked at the qualifications of camp staff who administered medications, the kinds of medication used by campers and staff, and the concerns raised by people who were responsible for the delivery process. The study results found that (a) people without training in medication management were giving medications to campers, (b) prescription medications brought from home often arrived at camp with incomplete information, and (c) medications from other countries were problematic (e.g., not FDA-approved, labeled in a different language). These points certainly raise a number of red flags for camp nurses.

A comment of particular interest appeared in Lishner and Bruya's last paragraph: "Parents and pediatric nurses might assume that a more sophisticated level of health care is being provided than actually exists" (p. 253). This statement referred to the researchers' observation that (a) people without medication training were involved in making medication decisions (e.g., trip staff) and (b) communication about medication practices at camp were not clear. Medication practices should be written in detail and shared so parents, physicians who do camp physicals, camp administrators, and the camp's healthcare providers have the same expectations.

Rudolf, Alario, Youth, and Riggs (1993) examined the age at which children were given or assumed responsibility for taking medications — and used a residential summer camp population to do so. While we question their research design, the researchers did note that children as young as nine years were already self-medicating. This observation may explain why so many children walk into camp health centers "knowing" what they want to take for their problem.

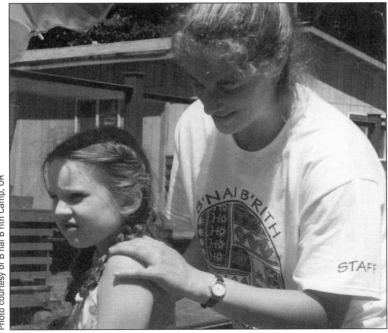

Photo courtesy of B'nai B'rith Camp, OR

Perhaps the best guide to medication management is Lishner and Bruya's book, *Creating a Healthy Camp Community: A Nurse's Role* (1994). Chapter 9, "Management of Medications in the Camp Community," includes a discussion about who should make decisions regarding medications, how to process meds on opening day (screening), handling inadequate information or inappropriate meds, determining "controlled possession," ideas for documentation, and management of medications on trips.

Regulations That Impact Medication Decisions

The regulations are specific to the state in which the camp is located. Pharmacy regulations, the Nurse Practice Act, the physicians' regulatory body, and regulations for ancillary providers (e.g., EMTs) used by the camp influence medication management decisions. In addition, regulations associated with the camp's license to function in that state may also influence decision making. Pharmacy regulations, for example, may preclude dispensing epinephrine in the camp's name but allow for dispensing it to a given individual. Physicians' prescription privileges enable them to freely work with medication, whereas an RN's practice is limited to those specific medications delegated through physician orders, such as the camp's treatment protocols, for use in a given situation. The bottom line is to research state regulations. Understand to whom they apply and under what conditions.

What Is a Medication?

From a camp perspective, "medication" refers to substances that people use either routinely or as needed to maintain their health and/ or to promote recovery from events of injury or illness. Medications may be for internal use, such as a pill, or for external application, such as a topical cream. In the camp setting, alternative remedies and vitamins and food supplements are usually considered "medication."

Location and Security of Medication

Most medications are kept in the camp's health center, a controlled setting where access is monitored by a person, such as the camp nurse, who understands when and why a particular medication is used. Medications, including refrigerated ones, should be in an area of the health center that can be locked.

While keeping all medications in the health center is generally sensible, some people need immediate access to their medication either to stop the debilitating effects of a particular condition or to maintain their normal life practices. Using Imitrex for migraine management is an example of the first situation, while carrying Lactaid for times when a lactose-intolerant individual chooses to eat something containing lactose illustrates the second. A practice that supports both these individuals and the need to monitor is the use of a "pocket pack." This is simply a one-dose supply of the necessary medication *which the person carries with them* to use when needed. Restocking a pocket pack keeps the client in touch with the camp nurse. Since it's a one-dose supply, the restocking contact provides the nurse an opportunity to assess the situation on an on-going basis.

Other exceptions to the proviso of keeping all medications in the health center include asthma inhalers used on a prn basis. Often called "rescue inhalers" by campers, these need to remain with the person. Some camp nurses permit the individual to carry the inhaler and then periodically check with the person to assess use and effectiveness of the therapy. Other nurses work with a staff member who, because of the way camp is organized, travels with a group of campers and can be relied upon to provide the inhaler when it is needed. Epinephrine is another medication that might be carried by an individual, especially someone with a known anaphylactic reaction. Depending on the individual and the situation, a client might carry his or her epinephrine.

In addition, topical medications used for acne control might remain with responsible older campers and staff. When inhalers and anaphylaxis kits are carried on the person, they should generally be kept in a fanny pack that zips closed. "Carried on the person" means exactly that — these emergency medications do not belong on the cabin shelf!

Practice Hint

Ask the camp director to explain how medications were managed the previous summer, especially those kept by campers and staff.

In essence, though, the expectation is that most medication is kept in the health center and monitored by the camp nurse, and exceptions should be limited. The key to making this work is developing a system that helps general camp staff identify which prescription medications have an "OK" from the healthcare staff to remain with the person. For example, a camp nurse could use an indelible marker to initial the medication container as a visual reminder to staff that the medication has been given an "OK" to remain with the individual. If a medication shows up without those initials, it's a cue to staff that the particular med and person using it should be referred to the health center.

Just because people carry a particular medication with them does not exonerate the camp nurse from monitoring the situation. People who carry inhalers, for example, should be periodically asked if they've had to use their medication and if its use has been effective. Support monitoring strategies by an occasional summary note on the individual's health record.

Sometimes staff medications are kept in a "staff only" area. It is possible to do this as long as the area is genuinely accessible only to staff. Discuss this option with the camp director before offering it to staff. And remember to assess staff for self-medication should they seek healthcare from the nurse.

Permitting an individual to carry or keep a particular medication means the nurse must appropriately monitor the situation. For example, a camper carrying a rescue inhaler should be asked every so often about use of that inhaler and the response documented. In addition, people who abuse this option should be placed back into the more routine practice of keeping medication in the health center.

Medication and Delegation

A person with appropriate knowledge about medications should be the one to make medication decisions. This is often a physician who, via label on prescription bottles or written treatment protocols, defines what medications are used and under what circumstances. A physician delegates medication decision making to a RN through treatment protocols which, in the camp setting, specify what medication the nurse may administer and under what conditions.

Note that "giving a medication" is different from making a decision about what medication to give. This is often the point where questions creep into the discussion because camps make use of personnel in addition to physicians and/or nurses. Wilderness first aid-certified personnel go on camping trips; a staff member may be asked to give routine, daily meds on the nurse's day off; an assistant in the health center is told to give a certain individual two ibuprofen every four hours until her cramps are better.

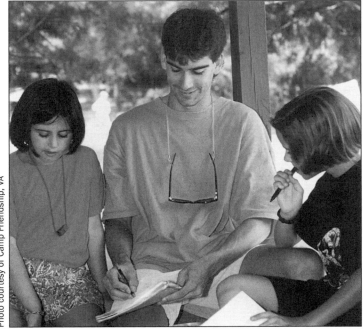

Photo courtesy of Camp Friendship, VA

From a nursing perspective, each of these circumstances brings professional delegation skills into action: assessing the ability of an adult staff member to carry out delegated instructions, providing clear directions regarding specific medications to specific people, and monitoring delegated tasks (e.g., checking completion of a med card or the return of empty pill envelopes or talking with people after the trip).

The delegation process, however, *does not* include assessment. Most Nurse Practice Acts quite clearly state that an RN retains the responsibility to assess situations and needs. Ancillary personnel may collect information, but it is the RN's task to make a decision based on what the information indicates. Here is where camp medication situations get tricky — especially for OTC meds. It's one thing for a camp nurse to determine a person's need for cold medication based on the results of an assessment and to direct an assistant to give the individual 60 mg of pseudoephedrine every four to six hours along with two acetaminophen every four hours. It's quite another to have an assistant carry out the assessment and, based on their findings, determine a medication choice.

Available information about nursing delegation is extensive. Camp nurses who delegate should understand this information. Consult the Board of Nursing if interpretive assistance is needed.

Most camp nurses do well with medication management. A greater concern occurs when the camp hires a "camp health manager" without medication education and then expects the manager to fulfill a job description that includes giving daily, routine medications as well as making decisions about the camp's stock medications. Today's camper and staff health profiles are complex. It seems reasonable, and the public would expect, that the camp would have a person appropriately skilled with medications if the camp includes medication management as part of its services.

Documenting Medications

There are a couple things to keep in mind that influence where and how medications at camp are to be documented. Some state regulations specifically direct a particular way in which health records must be kept; for example, use of ACA's Camp Health Log is cited by a few states. If this is the case, then all health records — including medication records — go there. This limits your options for record keeping.

Most regulatory bodies, however, do not describe a particular way or place for health records; they simply state that health records must be kept. In this situation, how one chooses to record information is then governed by the usual and routine practices of medical record systems: the record is unalterable, it shows date and time in a sequential manner, it records complete information, and so forth.

Many camp nurses record administration of prn meds on the individual's health record, whereas a special form is often created for routine, daily medications. This "daily medication record" is often based on the medication administration records used in hospital settings. The person's name, his or her med, and the order are written, followed by a series of small boxes that are initialed as meds are given on specific dates and at specific times. Records such as this should be filed as part of the camp's health record system and *be supported by a written policy setting forth the parameters for use.*

This last point is crucial, especially if multiple nurses work at a camp. A written medication management policy should clearly describe forms, detail how those forms are used, and delineate storage of medication records in relation to the total health record system.

Administering a camp's medication program is complex and warrants thorough understanding before a delivery system can be created. Consider the complexity of camper and staff medical histories and the increased use of alternative remedies, factor in a camp's schedule and the promises made to parents, and then develop a medication system that provides adequate assessment so the appropriate medication is given, adequate supervision so medication is appropriately administered, and adequate follow-up to assess therapeutic response.

Unlicensed Assisting Personnel: Their Role with Medication

The decision to dispense a medication is a delegated task from physicians to RNs via medical protocols. In assuming medication tasks, the RN retains — and cannot delegate — the responsibility to assess clients and make decisions based on that assessment. An assistant might help pass routine, daily medications; however, assisting personnel should not determine individual need for specific OTC or prescription meds. Assisting personnel should act on direction from the RN on a case-by-case basis. In using these helpers, the RN retains responsibility to monitor their actions.

Dispensing Medications

Daily medications are usually passed in one of two ways: (a) people receiving them simply come to the health center at the scheduled time or (b) medications are brought to an activity attended by everyone and dispensed there (e.g., at meals, after evening program). Regardless of the method used, you are responsible for seeing that those campers on a daily medication schedule receive the medication according to prescription order and/or parental request. If a camper forgets to come, you are expected to locate and get the medication to the camper.

Personal prn medications are generally dispensed when the individual requests them. You are cautioned to use your judgment and help campers accurately assess their need for prn medication. Under no circumstance should a prn be given merely upon request by a camper. You should verify the request. If strong doubt exists, a call to the parent may be needed. Document such instances in your notes.

With regard to staff, many camps assume that adults can accurately assess their own need for personal prn medication and will give these when the adult requests them. If you disagree with the adult's request, ask questions tactfully, but get an explanation. Continued disagreement should be documented and the rationale for your decision provided.

Medications stocked by the camp are dispensed based on your evaluation of the client. Use of stock medications is governed by treatment protocols issued by the camp's supervising physician.

Charting Medications

As in any other practice setting, medication that is administered for any reason should be documented. Documentation includes the following information: name of person, name of medication, reason for giving the medication, dose, route of administration, time of administration, therapeutic effect, and name or initials of dispensing person.

Record prn medication, both personal and camp-stocked, on the individual's health form as it is dispensed.

Daily medication may also be recorded on individual health records each time it is given or, as we said earlier, you may design a form — a Daily Medication Record (DMR) — and use it for charting daily medications. Such a record should be considered part of the camp's permanent health record and filed with those records at the end of the camp season.

■ Using a Daily Medication Record
(See Appendix F.)

1. Record all entries in black ink.
2. Use a new form for each session; label the DMR with the session dates/code. *Do not mix* people from one session with those of another.
3. Write the calendar date below the letter corresponding to the weekday of the session. The sample DMR begins with a Monday (Opening Day) but can be adjusted to reflect a specific camp's start day.
4. In the column labeled "Name and Medication Order," legibly write the legal name of the person getting the daily med followed by the medication order (name of med, route, dose, etc.).

5. Use the "Hr" (hour) column to record the time of administration. Coordinate medication passing with meals if possible.
6. Use the succeeding columns, each one dated, to document (initial) administration of the medication using these symbols:
   a. Your initials or an assistant's within a square indicate that the med was given as ordered at the date and time indicated.
   b. A circle within a square indicates the med was not given or was withheld. Document the reason for this action on the person's health record.
   c. A line (———) through the square indicates that the medication was not given because the person had not yet arrived at camp, had left camp, or started the medication when indicated on the record.
7. When a person self-administers (e.g., insulin, inhalers, sublingual drops), write the word "self" in the appropriate square.
8. The person who gives the medication is the one who signs off (by initialing the square) on the medication. The corresponding signature, credential, and initials should be entered at the bottom of the medication sheet by those whose initials appear on the form.
9. Monitoring each person who gets daily medication is important since medications are taken for a specific therapeutic effect. Occasionally ask each med recipient how he or she is doing. Know the untoward effects of the medication and watch for them. Chart the results of this evaluation process on the health form. Depending on the length of stay, it may be possible to do a summary note of this information when completing the Exit Note for the individual.

Ask the camp director what information parents were given about sending medication with their camper. This is no guarantee that those instructions will be followed. Contact the appropriate resource (e.g., parent, camp nurse supervisor, MD) if a question about a medication arises. NEVER give a medication that you question!

Refilling Personal Prescriptions

During the screening process on Opening Day, check personal prescription medications for quantity. There should be enough to last the duration of a person's camp stay. If a quantity is insufficient, call the camper's parents and alert them to the situation. They may want to refill the prescription themselves and send it to you, or have their physician call the camp's pharmacy (have the pharmacy's phone number available when you contact the parents) with a refill order. After asking the camp director, tell the parents how billing should be handled if the prescription will be filled through a local pharmacy.

Medication in First Aid Kits

In general, first aid (FA) kits should not contain medication. However, specific kits, because of their intended use, may contain certain medications. For example, trip kits are stocked with medication appropriate to the nature of the trip group and individual participant needs.

When you prepare an FA kit that includes medication, educate the staff who will use the kit about the medication, the parameters for its use, and how to document its use (most camp FA kits have a small notebook for this purpose). When the trip returns, review kit contents; note medication use and documentation.

Medication Errors

Talk with the camp director about the procedure should a medication error occur. Most camps handle these via incident report. It is usually the responsibility of the person noting the error to immediately bring it to the attention of the director and/or supervising nurse. The director is responsible from a liability perspective; consequently, it is important for the director and nurse to work through the situation together.

Obviously, the first concern is for the client and his or her safety. Assess the person. Contact either the prescribing physician or a physician at the camp's clinic. Explain what happened and follow the order given by the consulting MD. It is conceivable that both the prescribing MD and the camp MD should be consulted, particularly if an adverse effect is expected. Start documenting actions.

Also contact the camper's parents. Under no circumstances should this be neglected. The parents should be briefed about what happened, the health status of their child, and the follow-up action taking place.

Assuming the error was made by a person on the camp healthcare staff, this person generally should use the camp's incident report form to document actions as they occurred. Action from this point forward is a function of the given situation and is addressed on a case-by-case basis.

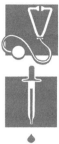

CHAPTER 9

First Aid Practices

Camp staff often have certification in first aid. If they function as first responders to camp emergencies, talk through your triage protocols since training agencies place emphasis on different elements. Also determine which first aid protocol is preferred by the camp and what is used for trips. ACA Standard HW-1 defines minimum expectations in this way:

- When access to an emergency medical system is within twenty minutes of camp or a trip group, a person with at least basic first aid and CPR certification must be with the group.
- When the camp or trip group is within twenty to sixty minutes of EMS, the credentialed person must be trained in "second-level" first aid and CPR.
- When the camp or trip group is more than sixty minutes away from EMS, a person with at least wilderness first aid and CPR credentials should be on duty.

FA kits are often created by the camp nurse for use by these and other staff when they respond to incidents as first aiders. Recommend that the scope of in-camp response be limited to coaching self-care since you are on site. Part of creating a FA kit includes the responsibility to (a) educate staff to use the kit effectively, (b) monitor

101

use of the kits, (c) replenish supplies, and (d) supervise usage documentation. First aid kit notebooks are often put with other camp health records at the end of the season.

First Aid Kit Documentation

Each kit should include a notebook within which the person providing care documents the situation and the action taken. At minimum, these elements should be recorded:

1. Date and time of incident
2. Legal name of individual
3. Description of signs/symptoms and incident that caused them
4. Description of first aid provided and/or coached
5. Signature of person who provided the care

Practice Hint

Have the camp secretary type the five FA documenting cues on labels, and then stick one to the cover of the small notebook contained in each first aid kit. This helps staff remember what to document.

First Aid That Counseling Staff Can Provide

Counseling staff are capable of meeting some basic health needs for campers. While major concerns are directly referred, items of less concern can wait for office hours. When a camper feels slightly ill or has a minor injury, staff can usually initiate care while the camper is still in the activity or cabin. By doing so, the camper feels "cared for" and interruptions are minimized. In no way does such care replace that which you provide; rather, it means the staff must decide if the injury/illness can wait until the health center is open or if the camper should have immediate attention. The following guidelines describe the parameters of that decision-making and care:

1. Camp staff may only coach the level of care for which they have been trained and is appropriate to their job. For example, a counselor with general self-care knowledge may coach a camper's

self-care for a bleeding mosquito bite but must refer a camper with greater healthcare needs.

2. Universal and standard precautions must be used:
   a. Gloves are worn when the potential to come in contact with someone else's blood or any other body fluid exists.
   b. People (children and adults) are coached to put on their own adhesive strips.
   c. A minimum fifteen-second hand washing with soap is required immediately after providing first aid.
   d. Campers and staff dispose of their own tissues in wastebaskets; staff who pick up potentially contaminated items must use equipment (e.g., a dustpan) to reduce risk and then must wash their hands afterward.
   e. CPR is provided only by designated people who must use face shields to minimize communicable disease.

3. Bleeding wounds that can be controlled by using an adhesive strip should be washed with soap and water, gently towel dried, and then covered with an adhesive strip from a first aid kit. People are coached to put on their own adhesive strips. Bleeding wounds that cannot be controlled with one adhesive strip must be referred to the nurse.

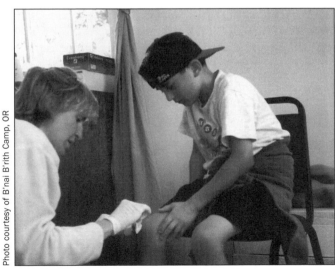

Photo courtesy of B'nai B'rith Camp, OR

4. While usually not life-threatening, headaches can be debilitating. The person suffering from one does not feel well and will not be able to perform optimally. This does not necessarily mean stopping participation, but it often means adjusting performance expectations. When campers complain of headache, move them to shade, let them relax (rub their shoulders), provide water, ask them to put on their sunglasses, and refer them to the nurse during the next office hour.

   Caution: Headache can be a symptom of larger problems. The nurse should be immediately contacted if headache is accompanied by vomiting, dizziness, and/or vision disturbance.

   Prevention: Headaches often can be minimized by adequate fluid intake, sufficient rest, activity adjusted to weather, and stress monitoring.

5. Cold symptoms (stuffy nose, cough, sore throat) can be miserable but are not life threatening. Staff should expect less than peak performance and encourage the person to conserve energy to avoid prolonging the cold. Offer the person water, a more sedate level of activity, shade, and more water. Remind the person to see the nurse during office hours. Expect colds to last seven to ten days; they are caused by a virus that can only be treated symptomatically. Cabin counselors should be certain campers with colds get adequate rest.

6. Bug bites are also irritating, but most can be avoided. Upon arrival, check the effectiveness of each camper's repellant (look for approximately 30% DEET), teach the correct way to use the repellant, and monitor its use. You should see "itchy mosquito bites" during office hours; they do not warrant an emergency visit. Check the itchy person's use of repellents.

Practice Hint

Impetigo can be started when dirty fingernails scratch irritating bug bites. Remind staff to have campers wash their hands — often! — and pay attention to dermal lesions.

Caution: International staff may experience greater swelling from their bug bites, particularly mosquito and spider bites. This is often a function of their bodies adjusting to the U.S. environment. Help international staff understand how to use their repellant (including how often to apply it).

Caution: It is normal for a person to swell at the site of a bite; it is not normal for swelling to occur other places. For example, a bee sting to the hand will cause swelling in the hand (maybe the wrist too) but should not cause swelling of the face.

Swelling at places other than the bite area requires quick referral to the nurse; DO NOT DELAY. The person may be reacting systemically — undergoing anaphylactic shock.

7. Homesickness (anxiety related to separation from one's normal support system) is felt in different degrees by different people, adults as well as kids. It can result in definite physical symptoms (headache, nausea, cramps, vomiting). If you suspect homesickness, *ask* about it! Homesick people need TLC and an opportunity to talk about their feelings. Children learn how to cope with separation just as they learn how to select friends; it is a developmental task.

   Homesickness care centers on the cabin counselors. The goal is to swing the camper's emotional affiliation from home to the cabin group. This can be accomplished in a zillion ways, but will generally require that he or she be allowed to vent emotions in a way that eventually relieves the stress without upsetting anyone else (including siblings at the camp).

   It is appropriate for the nurse as well as the camp director to be involved in more severe homesickness reactions. Conduct a conference with the camper, cabin staff, and any other staff member with whom the camper has bonded. Discuss the case; plan and implement an intervention. The key is to plan the care with the person's involvement in order to get her or him invested.

8. Use the RICE approach to treat most injuries (rest, ice, compression, elevation). The incident should be reported to the nurse. The nurse determines if the injury should receive further care.

9. Itchy rashes (e.g., poison ivy) can be washed with soap and water. They are not life threatening; the person should be referred to the nurse during the next office hours.
10. Most minor injuries (e.g., splinters, sunburn) can wait to be seen until the next office hour. Provide TLC and do not aggravate the situation (e.g., put a sunburned camper in the sun for an activity).
11. Counselors have priority care status! If they are hurt or ill, they need to seek care as soon as possible. Also, if a counselor who is caring for a camper's minor illness or injury is being diverted from the group's needs to the individual's need, the camper should be referred to the nurse. Counselors must put a priority on their group task.

Immediately refer to the nurse
- Bleeding not controlled by an adhesive strip
- Swelling at places other than the bitten area
- A camper who is throwing up (or threatening to do so!)
- A camper who looks sick (pale, tired, lethargic)
- Injuries needing a RICE approach
- Any injury to an eye or ear
- Emergencies

What Is an Emergency?

Campers define it differently from counselors and counselors define it differently from the nurse and the camp director will define it differently from everyone else! From a health services perspective, the "Five Bs" help define an emergency:

Barfing	Breathing
Bleeding	Burns
Bones	

Get the person to the nurse when these things happen!

CHAPTER 10

Communicable Disease Control

Communicable disease control is a priority in the camp community. Governing standards may regulate the amount of space per person, but that space is often minimal. Consequently, the population is an easy target for an epidemic response to illness. Campers and staff are frequently in close proximity to one another. They sleep in bunk beds; seating in most camp dining rooms is closer than that at home; and hand-washing areas are sparse.

As a result, using strategies to reduce exposure opportunities can make the difference between a relatively healthy camp and one complaining of colds, flu symptoms, and other syndromes. The nurse is often asked to monitor the environment and advise the camp's leadership staff when conditions warrant intervention of some sort.

General Control Practices

Several steps can be taken to minimize, perhaps even eliminate, communicable disease responses.

1. Thoroughly screen everyone, including staff and permanent employees, upon their arrival at camp. Follow the camp's screening orders with particular attention to asking about exposure to

communicable disease, attending to present illness complaints, and checking for head lice.

2. Insist that sleeping quarters follow the principle of maintaining the greatest distance between sleeping heads (top bunk has head at one end of bed, bottom bunk at the other).

Practice Hint

The rhyme "sneeze on the toes, not on the nose" helps everyone remember to alternate head placement when using bunk beds.

---

3. Orient staff and campers to good personal hygiene practices. Most will automatically think of keeping clean, but fail to recognize the importance of resisting a drink from a friend's soda can, the necessity of using their own brush and comb, and washing their hands with soap before table setting and meals.

4. Recognize dehydration and fatigue as contributing factors to headache, cold, and flu. Most participants, including staff, are not used to the program's demand on energy reserves. Suggest a modified schedule, an early bedtime or a morning sleep-in, when you suspect fatigue. Always look for ways to increase the camp's fluid intake. Make camp people more resistant to infection!

5. Rigorously pursue unexplained symptoms, especially if a body rash or GI upset occurs. It is far better to isolate people than to allow them to expose the entire camp population.

6. Occasionally, despite vigilance, a communicable disease erupts. A common example is chicken pox. When this happens, immediately isolate the individual. If there is any question about exposure control, contact the state department of health for advice. *Note: Immunocompromised people have special concerns when exposed to diseases such as chicken pox. Consult a physician so you can arrange appropriate prophylactic care.*

7. When a camper has a communicable illness that may involve being confined to bed and/or isolation for three days or more, talk with the camp director about contacting parents to get the camper home.

8. For purposes of control, define an "epidemic" for your camp and determine appropriate personnel to contact. (Some programs consider outbreaks of five or more cases with similar symptoms within a two- or three-hour span as an epidemic.)

9. Parents generally appreciate notification of communicable disease exposure. In conjunction with the camp director, a short, tactful, and to-the-point note can be designed for inclusion in a routing mailing. A sample follows:

A case of chicken pox was recently diagnosed at Camp Anywhere U.S.A. Chicken pox is usually a mild disease evidenced by a slight fever, malaise, and blisterlike skin eruptions that typically first appear on the trunk and scalp. The period of time from exposure to first symptoms is usually thirteen to seventeen days. If you have questions about _____ (the camper's) health, please contact (name, address, and phone number of camp's contact person).

---

10. Teach and use the techniques of universal precautions!

Concerning Deer Ticks, Poison Ivy, and Other Environmental Challenges

Camps are often located in areas where flora and fauna pose risks to campers and staff. Lyme disease, Rocky Mountain spotted fever, poison ivy/oak/sumac, red ants, scorpions, and rattlesnakes are among the more common challenges. Geography plays a part in what a camp nurse may discover at a particular camp, but so does the concept of emerging diseases. For example, West Nile virus has become a growing concern along the eastern seacoast.

Consequently, consider what may be a problem and make use of resources such as your state's department of health and the Center for Disease Control (CDC). CDC's Web site (www.cdc.gov) is particularly helpful and includes an international component for camps that have international staff.

Some camps have developed specific protocols to manage known risks. Discuss these with the camp director before campers arrive.

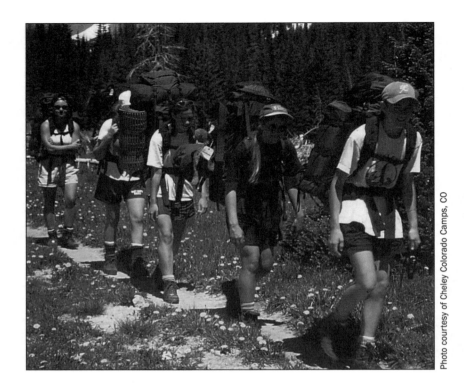

Photo courtesy of Cheley Colorado Camps, CO

Use local physicians to build needed clinical skills and/or fill in personal knowledge gaps about specific risks.

Global Issues and Communicable Disease

Today's campers and staff travel all over the world and many camps host staff and campers from other countries. As camps have gone global so have their health needs. Some concerns — like getting scabies from sleeping in hostels during world travels — are more of a nuisance and public relations issue than a *bona fide* health threat. But other diseases — such as the prevalence of tuberculosis in some countries — pose serious concerns.

Learn where international staff and campers come from; ask about travel history when clients present with unusual symptoms. Ask questions of the CDC or contact the state's department of health. Today's world is only getting smaller. Screen thoroughly, question inexplicable symptoms, and use isolation precautions if concerns exist.

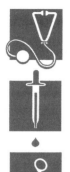

CHAPTER 11

Clinically Speaking

Camp nurses often wonder what types of illness and injury they'll see at camp. The answer is a function of such factors as:

- The age and health status of campers and staff
- The activities offered at camp
- The scope of the camp's risk reduction program
- The geographic location of camp
- The length of stay at camp
- The degree to which the camp attends to sanitation concerns
- The camp's investment in prevention rather than mere treatment

The best strategy for discovering what you might encounter is to look at last season's health records. These will help you determine not only the reasons for seeking health care but also when incidents were likely to occur. With a bit more investigation, it's even possible to determine if particular activities or camp locations were prevalent in injuries and who more often sought health care: males or females, campers or staff?

Regardless of the type of camp, there are components about clinical skills which impact all camps and, thus, the camp nurse.

"Treatment protocols" describes the care parameters — especially those pertaining to medication — expected by the camp's supervising physician and used by the camp nurse to meet general health needs of the camp population This differs from "standing orders," which describe care for a specific client. A camp's treatment protocols should be reviewed, revised, and signed by a licensed physician on an annual basis.

First, most camp nurses find that their clinical practice is helped when supported by treatment protocols from a physician. This is particularly important if the nurse is expected to use any medication (OTC or prescription). The use of medication is the domain of a physician; treatment protocols are the vehicle that enables a physician to delegate this responsibility to registered nurses. The protocols, which should be annually reviewed and signed (ACA Standard HW-11), must specify what medication to use in what situation.

Practice Hint

Use generic terms when referring to medications in the treatment protocols to have broad access to whatever brand of the named medication may be available. For example, refer to acetaminophen rather than Tylenol.

Sometimes camp nurses get so caught up in "giving medicine" that they forget how many nursing interventions do not rely on medication. Consider common human conditions — headaches, sore muscles, upset stomachs, sore throats, coughs, aching joints — and then recall all the nonpharmaceutical care approaches available to a nurse The camp nurse should consider coaching staff and campers in these self-care techniques:

- Relaxing techniques
- Drinking chamomile tea for nausea
- Drinking a glass of water and then another glass of water
- Sitting in the shade
- Using heat and cold
- Sleeping

- Breathing techniques
- Meditating
- Avoiding the discomfort's trigger (e.g., get out of the sun)
- Taking a cool shower or going for a swim
- Changing into more appropriate clothing

Clinical Tips from Experienced Camp Nurses

- There will be *many* sore throats: make plenty of gargle solution. Work diligently to reduce the threat of sore throats by addressing hydration status of campers and staff, preaching the benefits of frequent hand washing, and reducing the camp's fatigue factor. When a sore throat occurs, palpate the client's glands, monitor his or her temperature, note symptoms of upper respiratory infection (the common cold), know if he or she has a history of allergies. There are many reasons why a throat may be sore. The task is to determine that reason for each client and then develop a management plan that addresses that reason.

In clinical practice, always err on the side of caution. If in doubt, consult someone else.

- Know about the camp's flora and fauna threats and how to treat them Consider:
  1. Ticks: types, how to remove them, diseases associated with them, symptoms associated with pathology.
  2. Biting insects and spiders: what the bite looks like, the pathology associated with it, prevention techniques.
  3. Diseases of concern in the area: Hanta virus? Rabies? West Nile virus?
  4. Snakes: identification, how to treat their bite, avoidance behaviors.
  5. Poison ivy/oak/sumac: what the plant looks like as the camp season progresses, how the rash presents and how to treat it, at what point the reaction should be referred to a physician.
- Keep plenty of ice and cooling devices on hand. Fill med cups with water and tuck them into the freezer. Put a damp cloth in a

resealable baggie and place it in the refrigerator. Store extra ice in the camp kitchen's freezer.

- Stings usually increase as the summer wears on. Remove a residual stinger by scraping the edge of a stiff card over the sting site. Then mix baking soda with enough water to make a thick paste to place on the sting site. The baking soda paste draws the toxin, increases the sense of comfort, and keeps the camper busy while you collect whatever else may be needed (consider preparing the epinephrine).

- Review information about heat cramps, heat exhaustion, and heat stroke. Kitchen, waterfront, and maintenance personnel are most susceptible. Coach these people to drink lots of water all the time, take frequent breaks, and watch out for one another.

- Review anaphylaxis and the use of epinephrine and diphenhydramine in the management of an anaphylactic situation. People with known reactions typically carry their own epinephrine devices, but new allergies may be revealed at camp. Watch for the cardinal signs of a reaction such as swelling at a location other than the site of a bite, hives or a rash spreading over the body, a rising level of anxiety, difficult breathing and/or a sensation of a "thick tongue." *Know what to do!* This is truly a life-threatening situation that cannot wait for someone else to respond.

Practice Hint

Consider simply purchasing a vial of epinephrine for RN use; it costs much less than prepared epinephrine devices.

- There will be many slivers/splinters to remove so have a good pair of tweezers and a magnifying glass handy. Know where to find good lighting. Consider using a product like Mediplast for deeply embedded slivers. This salicylic acid pad, when placed directly over the place where the sliver went into the skin, hyperhydrates the skin (remember how skin looks prunelike when an adhesive strip is removed?) and, after a maximum of six hours, often "floats" the sliver to the skin surface.

- Remember that conjunctivitis can be a marker of a sinus or ear infection, so palpate the sinuses and use an otoscope to check the ears. Not all conjunctivitis is infectious, e.g., allergic conjunctivitis.
- Teach staff that any chemical substance — including bug sprays — getting into the eyes requires an eye flush lasting at least twenty minutes. To flush eyes, consider using an appropriate IV fluid, spiking the bag, and controlling the flow over the bridge of the client's nose. Attaching a nasal cannula provides a natural "bridge" for the nose and two "spouts" of water. Expect the client's eyes to feel dry for a short while afterward and monitor vision status. Don't minimize eye pain.
- Consider how children who tend to wet the bed will be managed. Perhaps the last counselor in the cabin at night can wake the child and take him or her to the bathroom. Know how DDAVP works and how to store it (it is available both in a nasal spray and pill form). Consider how to manage wet linen while preserving the dignity of the camper.
- Hyperventilation happens to overexcited people. Know how this presents and how to work with a hyperventilating person. Currently, using a paper bag is discouraged; simply calm and reassure the person (Thygerson, 2001). Clearing the room of other campers may help the hyperventilating camper focus on your suggestions.
- Consider spending time at an orthodontist's office before going to camp. Understand the basics of braces — how to remove a loose bracket; when to cut a wire that is poking into someone's cheek, and how to do it so the wire doesn't fly down the back of the person's throat; when *not* to cut a wire; how to put an elastic on a bracket.
- Consider taking a Wilderness First Aid course because:
  1. Some camps are more than one hour from definitive care, which is what determines the need for wilderness protocols (Forgey, 2001).
  2. Most nurses aren't very familiar with prehospital care, yet many campers and staff consider their nurse to be the equivalent of a call to 911.
  3. Critical thinking skills in emergency situations are developed in courses based on wilderness protocols.

4. These courses coach the use of common items to meet medical needs. Remember that not many camps have suction or oxygen on the wall.

Camp Emergencies

In spite of good planning, things can still go wrong. In fact, part of risk management is identification of anticipated emergencies and planning the camp's response system. Those situations for which most camps plan are

1. Lost campers
2. Aquatic emergency (observed drowning as well as suspected)
3. Weather emergencies appropriate to the camp's area (e.g., tornado, hurricane)
4. Catastrophic fire and forest fire
5. Death of a camper or staff member
6. Threat of violence
7. Abduction of a camper or staff member

Preparation is achieved through such measures as planned and rehearsed emergency drills, having qualified staff, and availability of necessary equipment and transportation. The principles that govern responses to any emergency situation apply in camp:

1. Evaluate the situation completely and as quickly as possible.
2. Do the simplest thing consistent with good nursing care.
3. Take care of the most important conditions first — maintain open airway, control severe bleeding, and prevent shock (ABC protocol).
4. Activate the emergency medical system if the condition is considered serious and/or make provisions to take the client to definitive care.

The camp nurse often has a role in these planned responses and the camp director will explain the role. In most situations, the nurse simply goes on alert while other staff focus on searching and caring for remaining campers. Any alert status should cause the nurse to gather supplies appropriate to the emergency in preparation for anticipated victims.

Effective response to emergencies can reduce the physical, psychosocial, and economic impact of trauma upon those involved.

Clinical Notes About
Common Camp Injuries and Illnesses

- These notes assume a normally healthy population; people with preexisting conditions require appropriate adaptation.
- Information is based on our experience and these references: Backer, Bowman, Paton, Steele and Thygerson (1998); Black and Matassarin-Jacobs (1997); Forgey (2001); and Neinstein (1996).
- The notes are not definitive; they merely illustrate what might happen at camp and describe some actions taken by some camp nurses.

■ Abdominal Pain

Abdominal pain is a common complaint among children and teens. It is often related to emotional distress, a change in food or in eating patterns, or constipation. These should be considered during the assessment. Assessment should include appropriate auscultation and palpation accompanied by a history surveying diet, elimination patterns, and activity. Severe or persistent abdominal distress requires competent medical diagnosis and management.

Common stomach flu or diarrhea without a high fever should certainly be monitored; it typically self-resolves. Administration of clear fluids is recommended. Persistent distress or recurring distress warrants referral to a doctor. Chamomile tea may be given to relieve nausea. Mild, nonspecific diarrhea can be treated with instructions to avoid foods that increase GI motility.

■ Abrasions

Cleanse thoroughly with soap and water. Remove contaminating material from the wound. If there is extensive tissue loss, especially around joints, consult the doctor regarding treatment. After cleaning minor abrasions, apply antiseptic ointment with dry, sterile dressings. Once sero-sanguinous drainage has stopped, keep the wound clean and appropriately bandaged.

■ Anaphylaxis

Some people experience a systemic reaction to certain insect bites or foods. They are often identified through the camp health form. It is your responsibility to interview at-risk individuals and obtain a history of previous reactions, including interventions needed. Record the information on the health form. Attempt to distinguish between a true anaphylaxis and simple intolerance to a food or an insect.

On the other hand, some people have no idea they may be sensitive to the point of experiencing anaphylaxis. An allergy may develop over multiple or prolonged exposures to an antigen. Be prepared: anaphylaxis can occur at any time in a susceptible individual.

Sample Treatment Protocol for Anaphylaxis Management

1. If the person is conscious, give 50 mg diphenhydramine immediately.
2. Monitor vital signs at five-minute intervals.
3. Prepare to use epinephrine: an adult dosage is 0.3 ml subcutaneously injected; a pediatric dose is 0.01 ml/kilo body weight injected subcutaneously. Prepare at least two doses.
4. Get transportation ready for immediate departure; establish contact with an MD or an ER. If anaphylactic shock is suspected, administer the epinephrine and transport the person to the emergency room. The person may improve while en route but keep going. Because epinephrine works for about fifteen to twenty minutes, perceived improvement may only be related to its action. Be prepared to administer another dose of epinephrine if the person's symptoms worsen.

When a person gets bitten by an insect (particularly bees, wasps, and yellow jackets), remove the stinger and apply cooling packs, keep the person quiet, and begin monitoring for symptoms of anaphylaxis (e.g., anxiousness; generalized swelling of the body, particularly in the face and throat areas; difficulty breathing; hives). A paste of baking soda mixed with water will be soothing.

If a person is known to be at risk for anaphylaxis and reports eating the causative food or being stung by the insect, initiate the camp's protocol for anaphylaxis management. Also do so for a person without an anaphylaxis history who, nevertheless, experiences symptoms.

■ Asphyxiation

Respiratory emergencies demand immediate action. Begin artificial respiration with nonbreathing individuals immediately. Continue until the victim revives or is pronounced dead by a physician.

Inadequate oxygen intake is panic-inducing as well as life threatening. The conscious person may need calming while you are monitoring respirations. Administer prn medication for asthmatic conditions. Document the number of times inhalants are used during an asthma flare. (See Appendix D.)

Note: This symptom may be part of an anaphylaxis reaction to an allergen. If such is suspected, contact a physician via phone and prepare to use epinephrine as ordered.

Unconscious individuals with depressed respiration must be continuously monitored. Support breathing with artificial respiration as needed. Contact medical assistance immediately. Try to determine cause by noting environmental clues (e.g., carbon monoxide inhalation, drug use). If environmental conditions warrant, remove the victim to fresh air.

Treat respiratory emergencies for shock. People who are overcome to the point of needing respiratory support must be examined by a physician.

■ Athlete's Foot

Symptoms include itching, redness, and scaling between the toes. There may be cracks and small blisters. Wash the infected area with soap and water twice daily. Dry thoroughly and apply appropriate antifungal per directions. Cover the foot with a clean sock and instruct the person to wear shoes that promote dryness (e.g., canvas sneakers). Monitor for infection. Instruct the client to wear foot protection at all times to prevent contamination of showers and cabin floors.

■ Burns

Minor burns — first degree and those second degree with little blistering — of the body and extremities should be cooled with water (not ice) for twenty to thirty minutes, and gently cleaned with soap and water to remove contaminants. Adaptic dressings may be applied and secured with roller gauze. Avoid bulky dressings because maintaining joint mobility is important Do not break blisters.

A topical antibiotic may be ordered for any first- and/or second-degree burn. Per treatment protocols, an analgesic may be offered to control discomfort.

Burns are severe when a large area of skin is involved (consider the "Rule of Nines" used in first aid protocols), when there is extensive blistering in the burn area, or when third-degree burns are present. Do not attempt to clean or debride the area. Any loose contaminant may be removed from the skin, but remember these burns are originally sterile and can be recontaminated by blowing on them or touching them with hands or nonsterile instruments. Follow these steps:

1. Cover the burn area(s) with sterile compresses wet with cool, sterile water or normal saline. If the burned area is extensive (i.e., greater than a single limb), use a clean, dry sheet to avoid contributing to hypothermia.
2. Treat immediately for shock.
3. Arrange appropriate transportation to the hospital or clinic.
4. Check the person's health form for tetanus immunization status.

Always seek medical care for burns on the face or genitalia or over joints.

Encourage use of a sun screen for all campers and staff before sunbathing, swimming, boating, and any activity that places people in the sun. Work to limit exposure to the sun. When possible, activities should be done in the shade. Common kitchen vinegar applied to the affected area(s) will help relieve the discomfort of minor sunburn.

■ Cardiac Emergencies

In general, the camp population is a low cardiac risk group. However, the possibility of problems exist at the waterfront and among specialized staff (e.g., maintenance personnel). Many camp staff have basic CPR skills and should be able to provide basic life support. But they rely upon the nurse for coaching and supportive care.

Cardiac cases demonstrate primary complaints of pain in the chest, arms, or shoulders and they show signs of shock with a weak pulse, pale face, and a cold sweat. Often anxiety and fear are present; denial of cardiac problems is common.

Allow the individual to assume a comfortable position (often a semireclining position). In all cases of suspected heart involvement, call the physician and/or activate 911/EMS. If respiration ceases, begin artificial respiration. If the pulse cannot be palpated, begin CPR.

Record blood pressure and pulse every ten minutes while the suspected cardiac client is in the health center. Ask about the person's history of previous heart problems. Follow these steps:

1. Treat for shock.
2. Elevate head and shoulders if breathing is difficult. If available, administer oxygen per order of a doctor.
3. Check the client for nitroglycerin; administer immediately if found.
4. Contact the MD; have past history available.
5. Transport as soon as possible.

As this book went to press, automated external defibrillators (AEDs) were beginning to show up in camp health centers. Follow the camp protocol regarding the AED in suspected cardiac cases.

■ Chest and Abdominal Injuries

Torso injuries are usually caused by blunt force and most commonly produce two types of injury: a contusion or an open wound.

Chest bruises and contusions can be very painful without showing much evidence of injury. Common complaints are pain when breathing, coughing, and moving. Campers who fall from top bunks may complain of these symptoms.

1. Keep the person warm and comfortable.
2. Severe chest injury with respiratory distress requires that all movement (including transportation) be under the nurse's supervision and access to a physician is initiated. Consider the mechanism of injury (MOI) for possibility of spinal injury and immobilize as appropriate.

3. Treat for shock. Record vital signs at appropriate intervals and monitor level of consciousness (LOC).
4. Cover open wounds with sterile dressings.

Deep, penetrating wounds of the chest may produce a sucking sound. This demands immediate action as the person will develop almost immediate respiratory distress. If a sucking wound occurs, apply a plastic dressing to seal all edges. Additional pressure is best applied over the site by hand or adhesive tape. Consider these clients to have deep chest damage and arrange for immediate attention from a doctor. Treat for shock and monitor for deviation of the trachea.

With abdominal injuries, give nothing by mouth. Consider bruises and knife wounds of the abdomen to have injured deeper structures. Arrange for a physician to see this person. Apply dressings as necessary to protect the wound.

■ Conjunctivitis

Ask if any contaminant has recently been in the person's eye since an abrased eye surface may initially present similar to conjunctivitis. People using contact lenses should remove them; eye makeup should be removed and discontinued until the condition resolves. Check the color of tissues in the conjunctival sac: What color is observed? Is there a difference in color between the two eyes? Assess for associated nasal symptoms. Could this be allergic conjunctivitis, which is indicated by a "cobblestone" appearance in the conjunctival sac? If you suspect allergies, give an appropriate medication per treatment protocols and monitor its effect.

Is yellow matter present in the tear duct area and/or along eyelashes? If so, begin warm soaks for ten minutes every three to four hours during the day (discontinue at night). Consult an MD if yellow matter, redness, or pain persists beyond twenty-four hours. Take care not to contaminate the uninvolved eye. Stress the importance of frequent hand washing and only using one's personal towel/washcloth to minimize spread.

Consult a physician or ophthalmologist for care. Advise the patient of the condition's potential for contagion; emphasize extreme care with cleanliness and material disposal.

■ Constipation

Assess history for adequate water intake, effects of travel (especially among international staff), change in diet, and/or taking time for elimination while at the camp. Auscultate and assess bowel sounds in all quadrants.

Advise the client to increase fluid intake and to eat plenty of vegetables, whole grain breads, and fruits while minimizing foods that decrease bowel motility. The person may need education regarding the effect of the camp schedule (e.g., taking time for a BM) and the diet on bowel habits.

Give medication per treatment protocols if these interventions are not effective. Consult a physician if impaction is suspected.

■ Contusions

Initially, cool compresses applied directly to the area may provide pain relief and minimize swelling. Most references advise applying heat to contusions only after eight to twelve hours have passed. If soreness and/or disability persists, or if there is suspected deep involvement (note MOI), contact the physician. Recall that soreness associated with contusion may be the result of cellular debris at the injury site. Gentle increase of vascular supply will gradually improve soreness by removing cellular debris.

Note location, size, and quality of contused area(s). Consider history for the possibility of abuse.

■ Dermatitis (Also See "Poison Ivy")

Many skin rashes appear in the course of a summer. Most resolve without complication and may do so without the source of irritation being determined.

A contact dermatitis should be considered if the presenting rash is localized. Play detective in an attempt to discover what may have changed for the person in question (new soap? different laundry process?). Remove contact with suspected items. Treat the rash symptomatically per treatment protocols; consider a Domoburo soak if the client is particularly bothered. Expect the rash to improve – but not necessarily completely resolve – within twenty-four hours of care. Consult with an MD if this doesn't happen.

A localized rash can also indicate bug bites, impetigo, pityriasis rosea, viral illness, or infestation by a mite (e.g., scabies). The rash may also be an irritation caused by rubbing against inner tubes, the pool's kickboards, or the harness used at the ropes course, etc. Consider the client's history and note associated symptoms such as runny nose, itching, or fever.

A dermatitis that is fairly prevalent over all body surfaces should cause you to consider an allergic reaction if the person has recently begun taking an antibiotic. Withhold the drug and consult the client's MD in this situation Also consider the potential for diseases such as chicken pox and measles.

Occasionally, a counselor or camp worker will think a skin condition is due to the work environment. Conduct an assessment, including a history with the suspected reactive agent and reference the chemical's material safety data sheet (MSDS). Refer this person to the doctor for consultation if appropriate.

■ Diabetes

Campers and staff who have diabetes should be interviewed by the nurse within twenty-four hours of their arrival. Consider using a "Diabetes Information" form (see Appendix E) at this time and, based on the information received, inform the appropriate personnel (e.g., cabin counselors, kitchen staff) as needed to support the person's diabetes care plan.

Since diabetes complicates wound healing, consult an MD when people with diabetes get injured. Observe and document the healing process in time increments no greater than twelve hours. Foot injuries in particular may need the attention of a MD.

A known diabetic who appears confused, has difficulty speaking, or shows other signs of being distressed (feels hungry or jittery or acts strange) may be experiencing a hypoglycemic reaction. The reaction is related to the body's low glucose and insulin levels and indicates a need for attention. This can progress to an emergency situation if not addressed. Feed the person a combination of short- and long-acting carbohydrates; usually a glass of milk or juice will help. If the person carries glucagon, administer it. Check the person's blood sugar at both the start and the end of hypoglycemic care.

Note: The use of glucagon may result in extremely high blood sugar levels for the next day or two.

If the person with diabetes is unconscious, follow the camp's treatment protocol to rouse him or her.

Consider talking with parents of campers who experience a hypoglycemic reaction; these families appreciate knowing of their child's experiences. Suggest that adults who experience a reaction contact their diabetic educator.

People who have diabetes and who experience febrile illness should be admitted to the health center for close monitoring of blood sugar. Insulin, fluid, and carbohydrate intake must continue to prevent diabetic ketoacidosis and dehydration.

■ Diarrhea

An isolated case of diarrhea is usually not serious. Typically, it is self-limiting and will subside within a day or so. Always stress the need for fluid (water) replacement during diarrhea episodes, and encourage a bland diet emphasizing carbohydrates, fats, and protein. Consult the doctor if diarrhea persists beyond two days or is accompanied by high fever or blood and/or mucous in the stool.

Episodes of diarrhea that occur in several people within a few hours of each other may indicate contaminated water or food sources. If you suspect this, immediately notify the camp director.

It is also important to realize that many people are lactose intolerant. Because camp foods may be unfamiliar, it is conceivable that a lactose-intolerant individual would get diarrhea because she or he ingested milk-containing items without realizing it. A dietary history should reveal the offending item and the discomfort will eventually resolve.

■ Dysmenorrhea

Allow the person to rest as needed. Use of a heating pad or hot water bottle may help relieve cramping as may exercise. Give analgesics per treatment protocols. Analgesics are most efficacious if given every six hours (rather than prn) during the twenty-four to forty-eight hours the pain is most bothersome. If this is a new experience for the girl, assess her level of understanding regarding menstruation and offer appropriate reassurance. Advise her to talk with her mother when she gets home for more help and advice. Be sensitive to the fact that menarche may be a special time between mothers and their daughters.

■ Earache

Assess for the associated symptoms of rhinitis, cough, and sore throat. Pain from enlarged nodes can also radiate to the ear.

Does the discomfort increase when the ear lobe is gently pulled? This is a classic indication of an outer ear infection and sufficient reason to keep the ear canal dry (so no swimming). Consult an MD. Do not rule out otitis media; it can exist concurrently with otitis externa. Once the inflammation has subsided, you can request preventive drops for the client's use after swimming and showering to prevent recurrence.

Is the ear discomfort unaffected by gently pulling on the ear lobe? Does the person have a history of a URI? Give medication per treatment protocol and hydrate the person. If you are skilled in doing otoscopic exams, assess the tympanic membrane and other structures. Consult an MD. Provide an extra pillow to enhance the client's comfort while lying down. Monitor temperature and offer a mild analgesic as needed.

■ Enuresis

Do not make an issue of this potentially embarrassing situation. Attempt to determine the cause for the bed-wetting. For some campers, it may be the result of deep sleep (overtiredness), fear of leaving the cabin at night to go to the latrine, or homesickness. Talk to the camper's counselor and work out some way to take care of the wet linen without causing embarrassment. If bed-wetting is new or is accompanied by urgency, frequency, or pain on urination, refer the client to the physician. Also consider calling home; some parents neglect to put this information on the health form.

■ Eye Injury

Injuries that involve bleeding from or around the eye must be seen immediately by a physician. Do not make an attempt to examine the eye or instill medication. Place a dressing over the injured eye and bandage both eyes without pressure.

Objects impaled in or near the eye should not be removed but bandaged to prevent further movement. Again, cover both eyes. Transport to an MD or ER immediately.

Removal of a contaminant from the eye begins with locating the irritating factor. Remove it with a sterile swab or flush the eye with sterile saline. Have a doctor see the person if the irritation cannot be removed.

A persistent sensation of a foreign body in the eye is symptomatic of a corneal abrasion and should be referred to an MD for evaluation. Remove contact lenses ASAP and keep them out until an MD approves continued use.

Follow these steps when dealing with an eye injury:

1. All injuries to the eye that cause bleeding must be seen by a doctor.
2. Prevent additional aggravation; do not even examine the eye if the physician will be available to do it.
3. Always bandage both eyes to control movement of the injured one.
4. Never remove impaled objects. Bandage to prevent additional penetration.
5. In cases where eyelids and/or surrounding tissue are contused or lacerated, apply a firm bandage to control bleeding and transport.

■ Fever

Persons with temperatures above 100°F. are usually admitted to the health center for observation and treatment. However, it is important to assess the person — is he or she, in fact, ill? Children in particular may run slightly elevated temps simply because of dehydration and/or fatigue and need amended schedules (e.g., rest hour in the health center) to support recovery. Do not minimize this care. Slightly elevated temps mean a person is more susceptible to further compromise.

If the person is uncomfortable (e.g., headache, ache in joints), administer an analgesic per protocol until the fever subsides. Force fluids (water). Attempt to determine cause while providing symptomatic relief. Contact the physician if a fever persists beyond 48 hours or if it goes above 102°F.

■ Fracture

Fractures are not always obvious and should be suspected when the mechanism of injury includes sufficient force to have caused a fracture. A suspected fracture should be immobilized. Keep the client quiet and treat for shock. Cover a bleeding area of an open fracture with dry, sterile dressings. Do not attempt to reduce fractures unless you are functioning with specific wilderness protocols for fracture management. Transport for x-ray diagnosis.

Suspected fractures of the back and neck must always be handled with care. Carefully consider the need to move any client with a suspected back or neck injury. Activate the camp's EMS; consider waiting to backboard until the local EMS responds. Work to stabilize the client by treating for shock, assuring an adequate airway and respiratory effort, and conducting a secondary assessment. If they are needed, the aquatic staff are usually skilled in the backboard process.

■ Headache

Headache is frequently disabling and can be a symptom of other problems. Many times, however, a headache is simply a result of fairly common human concerns: fatigue, homesickness, dehydration, tension, constipation, too much sun, or overindulgence in food. In each case, obtain a history to determine etiology. Take the person's temperature. Bed rest and an analgesic per protocol will often ease the discomfort.

Sustained discomfort, headaches that occur upon rising in the morning, or headaches that accompany neuro signs warrant contacting the physician. The combination of headache, vomiting, and a stiff neck demands immediate medical attention. Monitor blood pressure if the client is an adult.

Migraine headaches are characterized by a sudden onset of throbbing, severe pain that is often localized. Once they are established, migraines do not respond readily to bed rest and analgesics. Consequently, the secret to fairly expeditious control is to provide the person in the prodromal phase of migraine with analgesic per protocol and a dark, quiet, cool resting place. Obtain the patient's history and treat symptoms accordingly. Contacting the physician may be necessary if the individual doesn't respond to treatment. People with a history of migraine often have available a prn prescription medication.

■ Head Injury

Head injury ranges from mild to severe. Monitor the person, particularly noting the level of consciousness and/or nausea. It is not unusual for a person with a moderate head injury to vomit once and to have a moderate headache and some transient dizziness. Anything beyond that behavior (e.g., vomiting more than once) is suspicious and you should contact the physician.

1. Keep the person prone with head elevated.
2. Apply cold compresses to the bruised/contused area. Give nothing by mouth and administer no sedatives.
3. Do a full baseline neuro and vital sign assessment. If normal, continue to assess and record vital signs every ten minutes for the first hour, and then every fifteen minutes. Assuming improvement, taper per protocol.
4. Treat for shock.
5. Assess the client's LOC periodically (appropriate to the situation).
6. Keep unconscious clients under your direct supervision. Transport to the clinic/hospital immediately.

■ Heat Exhaustion

Symptoms of heat exhaustion include weakness, dizziness, headache, and nausea. The skin temperature is usually cool and damp, and the person usually appears quite pale. Treat by bed rest with the person's head lowered. Maintain the person's body heat and gradually rehydrate. It may take a day or two to rehydrate adequately. Heat cramps may accompany heat exhaustion. Give water at fifteen-minute intervals or until the patient responds favorably.

■ Heat Stroke

Give no stimulants to heat stroke victims. This is a life-threatening situation that may require hospitalization. It is usually an insidious illness, one that can build over a series of hot, humid days in people who work in fluid-leaching, hot environments (e.g., kitchen staff). People with heat stroke may appear quite flushed and dry. Their sweating mechanism is no longer effective. Move the person to a cool area. Remove and/or loosen clothing; consider wetting the clothing to cool the person. Lay the person down with the head somewhat elevated. Apply cold wet packs or an ice bag to the head. Force fluids (water) if able to swallow and give a cooling bath. Monitor vital signs. Consider the need for IV rehydration. Contact the doctor and monitor LOC.

■ Hemorrhage

Minor cuts/abrasions of the hand, forearm, and knees and over-scratched mosquito bites are the most frequent causes of bleeding. Such light bleeds are self-limiting and serve to naturally cleanse a wound. More extensive bleeding is best controlled by direct pressure, regardless of whether the bleeding is venous or arterial. Apply a pressure dressing by using a tightly folded towel, a roller bandage, or several sponges bound tightly over the wound. Elevate an injured extremity above the level of the heart.

Generally speaking, do not use a tourniquet to control severe hemorrhage; most severe bleeding can be controlled with pressure. The use of a blood pressure cuff to compress bleeders prevents considerable trauma to underlying nerves and muscles. Follow these steps:

1. Expose the wound.
2. Remove obvious contaminants.
3. Apply pressure as needed for bleeding control, but do not make a tourniquet out of a pressure bandage.
4. Maintain good aseptic conditions and treat the patient for shock.

■ Impetigo

This skin infection, caused by streptococcal and/or staphylococcal bacteria, characteristically appears as lesions that begin as small red spots at the site of a break in the skin (such as from rubbing the nose or scratching an itchy bite). The spots progress to tiny blisters that eventually rupture, producing an oozing, sticky, honey-colored crust. Consult a physician about your findings; usually a medication will be ordered.

Impetigo can be passed from person to person by direct contact. Consequently, teach appropriate hygiene and coach behaviors that limit transmission to others (e.g., hanging one's washcloth in direct sunlight).

■ Injections

People requiring injections are usually managed on an individual basis. Those who self-administer medications such as insulin and human growth hormone generally continue that practice while at camp, although such self-care is typically done in the health center where access to a sharps container and supervision can be provided. Assess clients who self-administer for capability and appropriate practices. Be sure to show them where to put their used sharps.

Contact the camp physician regarding allergy injections. Allergy injections are *not* usually given at camp unless adequate support to manage an adverse reaction is available. Consider doing allergy injections if these supports are in place:

- Oxygen is available in camp.
- Capability to start an IV is assured (supplies and an able provider are at camp).
- Epinephrine is available.
- A physician is present who can effectively manage a reaction.

■ Insect Bites

A local reaction to insect bites/stings includes pain and swelling at the site. Treatment consists of removing the stinger or insect, cleaning the wound with soap and water, and applying cool compresses.

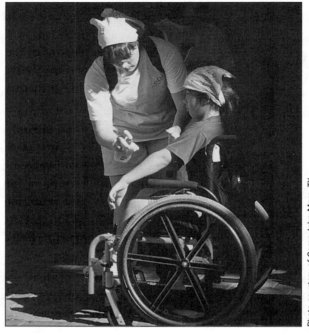

Photo courtesy of Camp John Marc, TX

Delaying the application of cold results in a more severe local reaction. Per protocol, give analgesics for pain and/or order an antihistamine to relieve itching.

Some people experience a systemic reaction to certain bites; they get stung on the arm and their whole body swells. This is known as an anaphylactic reaction. Refer to the orders specific to anaphylaxis. In general, when an at-risk person gets bitten, immediately apply cold packs and begin monitoring for symptoms of anaphylaxis (anxiousness; generalized swelling of the body, particularly in the face and throat areas; difficulty breathing; hives). Give an antihistamine and have epinephrine available.

Spider, deer fly, and red ant bites are particularly troublesome. The bite site may swell, become painful to touch, and get quite warm and red. Sometimes the person is not aware of having been bitten. While cool soaks appear comforting (consider prescribing a swim), nothing to date has been identified that truly changes the resolution process. Monitor the bite and expect resolution to take up to ten days.

■ Lacerations

Control bleeding to the extent that the wound can be exposed and examined. Determine if damage to deeper structures has occurred.

When the injury involves feet and hands, check range of motion to determine tendon involvement.

Check nerve involvement via a neuro assessment. If nerve damage is suspected or hemorrhaging cannot be controlled, have the physician see the client.

When the wound will be seen by the physician, the following is recommended:

1. Clean the wound only enough to apply a dressing.
2. Apply large amounts of sterile dressings with pressure for hemorrhage control.
3. Check with the physician about administering analgesics.

When deep structures are *not* involved, the following steps typically govern care of lacerations:

1. Meticulously clean the wound with soap and water.
2. When applicable, approximate the wound edges and bandage per protocol.
3. Cover the wound with a dry, sterile dressing. Splint the wound if necessary to protect it.
4. Redress all wounds that become wet or soiled.
5. Check the client's health record for tetanus immunization. Report to the doctor if one is needed. Immunization is usually considered current if inoculated within the past ten years unless the wound is highly contaminated. In that case, the physician may want to order reinoculation if five years have elapsed.

■ Nosebleeds (Epistasis)

Apply external pressure to the soft tissue just below the bridge of the nose and have the person sit or lean forward quietly until the bleeding stops. Check blood pressure. If bleeding is not controlled within twenty to thirty minutes, consult a physician.

■ Pediculosis (Head Lice)

Lice are seldom seen without magnification. Pediculosis usually presents with complaints of itching scalp or visualization of "nits," which are clusters of louse eggs. Without magnification, nits appear as tiny translucent lumps firmly attached to hair strands and rather close to the scalp.

Many camps have a "no nits" policy. In other words, individuals with head lice and/or visible nits must be treated and all nits removed before continuing their camp experience. Ask the camp director about the camp's head lice policy. This is especially important to know when a case is identified on Opening Day. It is certainly preferred that a parent treat an infested camper, but sometimes parents aren't present by the time campers go through the health screening process. In these situations, it is often the camp nurse's responsibility to supervise the treatment process.

> ### Practice Hint
> Some camps train a team of people — either staff members or people from the local community — to treat head lice and remove nits. The "Nit Pickers" are called when a case of head lice is identified at camp.

There are many treatment protocols for coping with head lice. One of the more common begins treatment by mixing one cup of common vinegar with one cup of lukewarm water. The individual's head is doused with this mixture and allowed to air dry. This solution softens lice egg casings, making them more permeable to penetration by the treatment chemical. After drying, treat the infested person's head with the selected pediculocide per directions and treatment protocols. Follow directions meticulously, including the instruction to comb through the hair and manually remove nits.

Linen and clothing (including hats and hair items) are usually treated by washing them in very hot water and then bagging the items and setting the bags aside for a few days.

The prevalence of head lice has increased over recent years and there is suspicion that the louse may be developing resistance to routine treatment. As a result, diligently screen heads upon arrival (of both staff and campers) and thoroughly reinspect a treated head on days three, six, and ten following treatment. Remove visualized egg casings. Retreat the head if lice are seen and/or if the number of egg casings seems to be increasing.

Since initial screening may miss an emerging case of head lice, consider rechecking the heads of people who remain at camp for more than two weeks. Also remind staff to note campers who may be scratching their heads more than normal and refer these campers to the health center for a head check.

■ Poisoning

Check the container for the appropriate antidote and administer it per instructions. Call the Poison Control Center for advice. Be prepared to use ipecac if directed to do so.

■ Poison Ivy, Oak, Sumac

One of the more common skin irritations may be poison ivy, oak, or sumac. The characteristic rash is caused by the plant's oil, urushiol (yoo-ROO-she-ol), penetrating dermal cells. Wash suspected cases with rubbing alcohol followed by soap and an extensive water rinse. Treat established cases per protocol. If results are poor, contact the physician. Severe cases may require systemic steroids and should be seen by a physician.

Calamine lotion or domoboro soaks are sometimes used for symptomatic relief. Domoboro soaks tend to be especially effective for extensive reactions on feet, legs, hands, and/or arms. Tell the client to wash contaminated clothing in hot, soapy water to remove the causative oil. Remember to assess the client's bed clothing for contamination with urushiol.

On occasion, a staff member (e.g., maintenance) may need to go through an area of poison ivy/oak/sumac to accomplish a job task. Consider having the person apply one of the barrier creams that are currently available to reduce, if not eliminate, the potential for reaction. Then have the staff person wash exposed skin with rubbing alcohol when done with the job and remove clothing carefully so the oil is not inadvertently spread.

Practice Hint

Read Hauser's book, *Nature's Revenge* (1996), to learn more about this common camp plague.

■ Ringworm

If a red ring (from which the fungus gets its name) is observed, contact the physician. Medication is usually applied to the affected area(s) three times daily. Improvement should be seen within a week, with no new red rings cropping up. Contact the physician again if the lesion does not respond to the medication. Address communicability controls with the client.

If a camper goes home with ringworm, advise parents to continue treatment until the lesions are completely gone. This may take as long as four to six weeks.

■ Shock

Shock is a condition in which the blood fails to maintain normal circulation throughout the body. It can be related to loss of body fluids, massive infection, CNS or spinal cord trauma, or cardiac decompression. Although its underlying cause can be obscure, shock almost always accompanies serious injury and may develop from minor injury, extreme nervousness, and/or fright. The most common symptoms are marked weakness, cool pale skin, perspiration (cold sweat), dizziness, a weak and rapid pulse, and nausea. Vomiting is sometimes experienced, too.

Every injured person should be treated for shock even though the signs may not be noticed right away. Shock may not develop immediately; symptoms can be delayed for several hours. Because of this gradual onset, it is easier to prevent shock than it is to control it after the symptoms appear.

Manage shock as follows:

1. Maintain the patient's body temperature. Keep the person dry, lying on his or her back or left side. Elevate the feet unless you suspect head injury and the person has difficulty breathing, or if the person complains of pain when the feet are lifted. Avoid unnecessary and rough handling.
2. Administer nothing by mouth to unconscious clients.
3. Monitor and record vital signs every ten minutes for the first half hour, then every fifteen minutes for the next half hour. Continue to monitor as needed or directed by the physician.
4. Medication for pain relief must be ordered by a physician.
5. Notify the physician as soon as practical if the person's response to this treatment is inadequate. Update the history by phone. Include vital signs, a description of the incident, and any history that might be a contributing factor.

While people expect shock in identified victims, it can also occur among bystanders. Perhaps someone has just seen a sibling injured or a counselor is feeling particularly anxious about the "supervision" she or he was supposed to be providing. You may be focused on the identified victim, but instruct other staff to look for shock reaction among others.

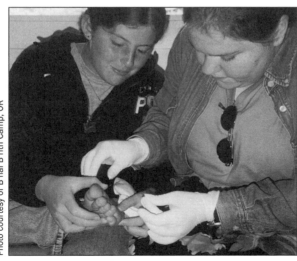

Photo courtesy of B'nai B'rith Camp, OR

■ Slivers, Splinters

Slivers always carry the risk of infection. Superficial slivers can be removed with a sharp, pointed splinter forceps. Sometimes a magnifying glass is helpful. Following this, the wound should be cleaned with soap and water, and dressed with antiseptic ointment per protocol and an adhesive strip. More deeply lodged, not easily accessible slivers may respond to the application of a small disk of Mediplast per protocol to the splinter entry site. Secure the disk with an adhesive strip for a maximum of eight hours and then remove. Any splinter that has not moved to the skin's surface within this time may need attention by a physician. Tetanus immunization status should be assessed in all of these cases.

■ Sore Throat

Visualize the throat and chart observations. Assess for nasal drainage related to URI or allergies; postnasal drip can irritate throats, as can yelling and singing loudly. If soreness is related to nasal drainage, give an analgesic per protocol to increase comfort and consider giving an antihistamine to minimize drainage. Saline gargles four times a day may provide comfort and will be most comforting if done just prior to eating. Explain to the patient that resolving a common sore throat may take a few days. Adequate rest and hydration are important to resolution.

Check the patient's temperature. An elevated temp may indicate several things, among them the early stages of a cold, viral pharyngitis, dehydration (which can make a sore throat feel worse), mono, or potential strep. Temps related to URI are generally subnormal. Monitor and chart temp every eight to twelve hours while the sore throat persists. Also note the individual's age, assess for tender nodes along the jaw, and observe the tonsils for size, color, and presence of exudate.

Consider requesting a strep screen if:

- There is history of exposure to strep (incubation period is usually one to three days) or the person has a significant history of susceptibility.

- There is *no* history of a URI.
- Onset was sudden and accompanied by fever, headache, and/or abdominal pain.
- Tonsillar exudate or petechiae on the palate are noted.

Some areas of the United States culture every sore throat; consult the camp's physician for a recommendation. If you suspect that a camper's parent may assume that a culture is "routine care," inform the physician.

A person with strep throat is considered contagious for twenty-four hours after starting antibiotics. Mode of transmission is direct or intimate contact with carriers; it is rarely by indirect contact through objects or hands. Explosive outbreaks (e.g., more than four cases from one cabin group) should be investigated for breaks in the camp's communicable disease control behaviors.

■ Sprains

A sprain results from stretching or tearing a ligament. The most frequent site is the ankle and the most common symptoms are pain, swelling, and discoloration. It is often difficult to tell a sprain from a fracture, so you should treat the injury as a fracture if there is any question.

The "Ottawa Ankle Rules" have been validated with adults and should be useful for teens. According to this, an x-ray is indicated if the client is unable to spontaneously bear weight (defined as four steps without assistance — even with a limp) within the first hour after injury or if point tenderness exists at the posterior edge of either malleolus or at the base of the fifth metatarsal.

If you suspect a sprain, ice, compression, elevation, and use of crutches will help to reduce swelling. The wrap should cover the spaces around the malleoli where the ligaments are located. To do this effectively, place a U- or donut-shaped pad around the malleolus before wrapping with an elastic bandage.

> **Practice Hint**
>
> If placing a person on crutches, remember to size the crutches to the person and teach crutch walking. Document this training. Also show the client how to check the crutches' wing nuts for tightness.

Rehab should begin as soon as the acute pain is gone. Range of motion exercises — such as getting the person to trace capital letters in the air with his or her foot — are good as well as going for a swim. The person with a sprain should be encouraged to bear weight as soon as the joint can be effectively supported with an ace bandage. If discomfort persists, refer the person to a doctor.

Use cold packs and splint if a finger, toe, or wrist is involved. Give analgesics per protocol. Symptoms usually subside in two to three days.

Severe sprains result when the ligament is stretched sufficiently to produce a tear in a portion of it. There is greater swelling, more tenderness, and considerable pain as well as discoloration due to hemorrhage. These sprains should generally be referred for medical assessment and are usually so swollen that wrapping is ineffective until some twenty-four to forty-eight hours postinjury. The injured area should be cooled until the wrap is applied. Once wrapped, the support should be maintained for two to three weeks.

A third-degree sprain results in a torn ligament and must be diagnosed by x-ray. This sprain requires complete immobilization for four to six weeks. It is typically more disabling than a severe sprain because of undertreatment. These sprains must be seen by a physician for prompt and proper treatment.

■ Strains and Muscle Spasms

If the person's symptoms are severe, keep the client on bed rest until seen by the physician or until you receive orders by phone. Mild cases of muscle strain and spasm usually respond to analgesics per protocol, massage, and external heat (e.g., hot water bottle, heating pad). Severe strains more commonly respond to cool-packs until it is convenient for the physician to examine the patient and prescribe.

■ Toothache

Administer a mild analgesic per protocol. The person should rinse his or her mouth with saline after eating. Persistent pain indicates the need for a dentist. Tell a camper's parents if their child experiences a toothache.

A fractured or displaced tooth requires immediate dental care. With minimal handling, place an avulsed tooth back in the socket, and have the person hold his or her tongue against it, or place it in milk for transport to the dentist. For optimum success, reimplantation must typically occur within two hours (and even that's no guarantee).

Pain from a broken tooth can be alleviated by coating the tooth with wax for braces until the person can see a dentist.

> **Practice Hint**
>
> The book, *Physician's Guide to Dental Emergencies* (Arizona Department of Health Services, 1998), explains dental situations and provides tips for field response until a dentist is seen.

Unconsciousness

The cause of unconsciousness can be obscure and symptomatic of another problem such as diabetic coma, fainting, excessive drinking, inhalation of toxic fumes, head injury, electric shock, or drugs. Still, try to determine the cause. Move the person only as necessary to achieve a physiologically improved position (e.g., elevate the legs for a simple faint). Monitor and record vital signs, and treat for shock. Check for Medic Alert identification. Contact the physician regarding *all* unconsciousness — even short term.

Remember: *If the face is pale, raise the tail; if the face is red, raise the head.*

■ Upper Respiratory Infections (Including the Common Cold)

Colds are a common complaint. If an individual's temperature is 100°F or more, consider admitting the person to the health center. Because of a cold's viral nature, treatment is symptomatic per camp protocol. Monitor vital signs and record all treatments.

Consider consulting a physician if symptoms are not improving after seven to ten days and/or if fever above 100°F persists over forty-eight hours.

Often sore throats are a precursor to other cold symptoms. However, if a sore throat is accompanied by a rise in temperature or remains resilient to treatment, strep infection must be considered (see comments under "Sore Throat"). Contact the physician or follow camp protocol to arrange for a throat culture.

While the common cold can certainly include a cough and congestion, the potential for bronchitis, sinusitis, asthma flares, pneumonia, and other illness exists. Auscultate the lungs and make note of sounds that differ or change. Monitor the person's temperature. Note color of sputum and any nasal drainage. Continue to hydrate the person and assure adequate rest.

It should be reasonably expected that people with a common cold recover without complication. URIs that evolve into sinusitis and other illness indicate greater debilitation. In these situations, determine if the client is, indeed, getting adequate rest and fluids and eating sensibly.

CHAPTER 12

The Psychosocial Domain and Camp Nursing

Jerry was on the cabin porch with his counselor, trying hard not to cry. It was evening on Opening Day; everyone was supposed to be in bed. "I don't know anyone! This place is so strange. I don't like swimming in a lake! I can't find my flashlight and it's too dark around here and my bug spray doesn't work! I want to go home — now!"

Nancy slunk into the health center, her face set in anger. It was the third day of camp. "I can't do this! I don't like it here. I hate my bunk mates and I need music when I go to sleep. No one told me it would be like this!"

Joe's counselor grabbed the nurse after lunch on the fifth day of camp. "You've got to help me. These kids are driving me crazy! They were perfect those first couple days, but now they won't cooperate — the cabin is a mess! They get on each other's case and they're picking on Joe all the time! He's driving me crazy too. He talks constantly and he can't sit still. I know he's ADHD but can't we give him more medicine?"

These scenes conjure all sorts of memories from experienced camp nurses. In fact, many camp nurses consider their work with physical concerns secondary to a connection with the psychosocial domain of campers and staff. Cleaning and putting a bandage on a wound is easy; having the person feel cared for during the process is trickier.

How does a camp nurse effectively connect with campers and staff? In other practice settings, nurses are often valued by how quickly and efficiently they can accomplish tasks. Starting an IV painlessly, inserting an NG tube without gagging the client too much, doing eight bed baths in an hour, and getting medications to everyone on time may define nursing care in some settings. Such is not the case at camp.

Clinical competence is certainly important, but camp nursing care is much broader. It includes behaviors that communicate to campers and their parents, staff, and camp administration that the nurse is interested in the people with whom she or he works. This kind of interest isn't defined by clinical competence; it's enhanced by caring behaviors such as:

- Consulting with parents about their camper's concerns
- Attending staff meetings and contributing to the total camp program
- Strolling around camp, talking with this activity head or that camper
- Keeping the director informed about staff and camper health without being asked
- Getting involved with a camp activity or two outside the health center
- Smiling; having an upbeat, yet genuine, can-do attitude
- Learning and singing camp songs
- Getting to a few campfire programs; maybe even participating in a skit
- Being comfortable with "clean dirt" as a health concept
- Eating meals with campers and staff
- Making good decisions, not merely popular ones

A dynamic tension exists between what a nurse intends to convey and what is actually perceived by the other person. This distinction is often captured by attending to communication skills. Effective listening, appropriate body language, and making reflective responses do more for campers and staff (not to mention the nurse's public image) than one would imagine!

The health center is a safe place for children when they need to cry. Tears shed in the company of the nurse might be considered socially acceptable. The nurse must take care that the crying does not get out of control and that the child doesn't use the empathy received from the nurse as a mental crutch. Children often behave as though the nurse were their parent. A transfer of feelings may benefit the child, but it can result in a "clinging vine" for the nurse. Sometimes the nurse needs to define the parameters of emotional expression. The camper's involvement in the camp program and with peer groups is his or her key to successful coping.

Consider the World from Which Campers and Staff Come

Most campers and staff come to camp with the intention of enjoying activities, working together, and striving for great outcomes: increased self-confidence, enhanced self-esteem, and improved social skills. But for some — like Jerry, Nancy, and Joe's counselor — something else happens. Then the dream of what camp might be is threatened; sometimes it never does become reality.

Campers and staff go through a physical preparation for camp; they pack their bags and give friends stamped envelopes to assure frequent letter writing. They also go through an emotional preparation. For some, the preparation and anticipation matches what they actually find at camp and then the transition generally goes fine. But others aren't so lucky. Their expectations differ, sometimes significantly, from what they experience or fail to experience. Then we get the Jerry, Nancy, and Joe's counselor situations.

The world of camp is different from the "other world" out there. Camp, a child-centered and nature-loving environment, is nurturing. Yet it can also be quite wearing. Those camps that clearly articulate the difference, tell people about the distinctions ahead of time, and identify strategies to help cope with the differences, contribute mightily to everyone's emotional well-being.

For example, in the outside world, children and young adults are taught never to talk to strangers, take anything from a stranger, or go to an unfamiliar place alone. Young people diligently use a set of survival skills suited to doing well in their home environment. Then one day, parents — the very people who work so hard to instill those survival skills — take them to camp. The parents drive away, leaving the young by themselves in a strange place with strange people and the admonition to "do as the camp director tells you." And we wonder why kids short-circuit?

The outside world wallows in technology: cell phones are in hip pockets, pagers are clipped to belts, Palm Pilots are tucked in book bags, and e-mail is preferred over snail mail. Campers and staff are tuned in, turned on, and moving! Then they arrive at camp and it all gets turned off or turned away. They're unplugged. They may become a bit unglued.

Consider the Camp World

In an effort to promote health, consider and address the distinctions between the worlds of home and camp. By doing this, people — campers and staff — have the information they need to shape an adjustment process. The camp health service could coach these responses by purposefully articulating the distinctions and discussing strategies to bridge the differences. For example, in selecting school-year activities for their children, parents often choose a program because it meets criteria such as being accessible to them "in case something goes wrong" and in close proximity to tools like telephones for "when you need me, just call" strategies. These criteria are not always relevant when it's time to go to camp, yet camps and parents rarely discuss this. As a result, parents rarely discuss it with their children. So the camper assumes that the operating principles are the same: parents are "reachable" and a phone is readily available.

Oops! The kids need to be clued in. That task may fall to the nurse, especially when a counselor brings a homesick child to the health center. Campers need to be told that camp is a safe place, a place where they go by themselves because self-sufficiency is a desired result. They need to know that it's okay and safe to interact with the "strangers" at camp even though it isn't okay to do so in other environments.

A camper's emotional readiness is also boosted when he or she understands that community living as a cabin group is quite different from having a bedroom at home. First of all, cabins are often shared with eight or more people. That certainly far outdistances the occasional sibling who might share the room at home. And while falling asleep to music from the stereo may happen at home, the camper is more likely to encounter snoring in the cabin.

In addition, the role of a camper's bedroom changes when they come to camp. Many young people use their home bedroom as an oasis, a place of solitude, and a great decompression zone after the fray of the day. This is particularly true for many teens. But camp bedroom space isn't like this at all. Finding an "alone spot" and keeping it that way takes skill! For those who need privacy or more significant quiet zones, camp life can be a significant challenge!

What About Staff?

Staff often have a different perspective of camp than campers. There's a certain thrill that goes with telling college friends that one is going to spend the summer working at a camp. Unique and risky activities take place and the job has a high social component, while conferring great responsibility to its staff. Working at camp can be a real rush, one that feeds into the young adult's developmental needs for risk taking and skill building. The staff members' preparation for coming to camp certainly includes thinking about themselves in this camp role — often in an idealized way. Once they arrive and begin working with campers, the work of group formation and maintenance — an often neglected topic during orientation — quickly becomes reality. That's when comments like the one from Joe's counselor are heard.

Staff may need to talk about what it means to be on duty 24/7. You can help by listening and by discussing how to massage time to meet personal needs, how to blend personal needs into the fabric of camp, and what to do when private time one was counting on must be used to care for a homesick camper. It's the day-to-day coaching of these skills that makes a difference.

A Word About People
with Mental Health Challenges

Campers and staff coping with emotional health concerns obviously have particular challenges. These individuals may not tolerate change very well and often do better when informed about changes well in advance. They also tend to have a smaller and more sensitive window for tolerating frustration. They, in particular, need to understand how camp differs from their at-home world before arriving at camp.

With preparation, this group often does well during its first few camp days. Then, about day four, it hits. The excitement of new people and places gives way to the tedium of living with cabinmates in a confined space. Energy used to screen the constant barrage of camp excitement begins to flag. Tolerance drops as fatigue sets in and simple things, like waiting in line at the dining hall, become a staging area for disintegration.

How can one reduce the potential that a well-designed camp management plan for such a person will fall apart? One way lies in building time into the person's day for unwinding and designating a place for that to happen. Today's youth have access to private spaces and time alone; for many, their bedroom serves this purpose. They come home from whatever the day presents and disappear into that space where they may use any of a number of strategies to unwind: listen to music, flop on the bed, strum a guitar, or sing as loud as possible.

When they move into camp, their private places disappear in favor of the cabin group and risk-reduction strategies such as "adequate supervision." Yet the need for occasional solitude may remain quite strong. Moments alone are all the more important if one has AD/HD and is using extra energy to screen extraneous noise and activity. Quiet, reflective moments are important if one has depression and needs time to process what's been going on. Privacy is important if one is coping with Tourette syndrome and has to express the idiosyncratic behaviors so diligently suppressed during the day. It's important if one has Asperger's disorder and just wants to escape the hoopla that others seem to thrive upon.

Discover where and when in camp people can be alone and then work with both campers and staff to use those places appropriately.

It's a real challenge to articulate the psychosocial differences between home and camp and then design strategies help both campers and staff during their camp experience, but it is also deserving of nursing attention. The holistic approach that characterizes camp's attention to youth means that camp nurses must see beyond the adhesive strips and Tylenol to the more fundamental health needs of campers and staff.

The health center is often a place where campers and staff who are coping with psychosocial issues go for help. In actuality, it isn't the health center that draws troubled people; it's the nurse. This is especially true when the nurse is perceived as a caring and approachable person who gives others a sympathetic hearing.

There are also typical situations when the advice of the camp nurse may be sought. Naturally, for the most part, this advice has a health basis. How often the nurse's advice is sought is a function of two broad factors: (a) the number of times a situation needing intervention occurs, and (b) the comfort felt by others in talking with the nurse. It is the latter that must be carefully managed. The nurse should strive to remain available and concerned about everyone. This approachability factor is influenced by others' perceptions of the nurse's reliability, responsibility, judgement, knowledge, and ability to maintain confidentiality. Document nursing interventions related to psychosocial needs.

Homesickness (Separation Anxiety)

Homesickness is a type of anxiety reaction that some people experience to varying degrees when they are separated from their usual support systems. It can affect anyone, children as well as adults. People tend to be more susceptible to homesickness in relation to the number of changes they experience at camp. The food, activities, sleeping areas, noise levels, and constant presence of other people are very different from most home environments.

People show symptoms of homesickness in different ways. Some express the anxiety by somatizing it: they may get headaches, feel nausea, vomit, and/or have generalized aches and pains. Some recognize the symptoms as homesickness and say so. Others may express the anxiety by becoming discipline problems or withdrawing from activity around them. This wide range of possible reactions is what can make homesickness difficult to identify.

A wise nurse realizes that people feel secure with routine. Moving to camp drastically changes routine and feelings of insecurity may result. In longing for the security of their home routine, some people cope in appropriate ways (e.g., getting teary-eyed when a letter from home arrives); others handle it inappropriately (e.g., prolonged crying, refusing to participate). Acknowledge and support appropriate coping responses and help people who are having trouble. The homesick person needs to identify the homesickness and then try a variety of ways to handle it.

Sometimes homesickness begins before the person even leaves for camp. Parents and well-meaning friends say things like: "Don't get homesick," or "I don't know how we'll get along without you," and "Who will feed your dog?" They may inadvertently give double messages: "Don't worry. You won't get homesick. And if you do, call me." These people may be genuinely concerned but not realize the impact of their casual statements. The camper may begin to think that the family can't get along without her or him, that it is unacceptable to feel homesick, and that the dog really won't get fed. No wonder they feel anxious at camp!

Reassurance usually helps. Denying the problem does *not* help — "Oh, you're just a little homesick. You'll get over it" — because the individual is already concerned. It is important to acknowledge the person's concern and explore its nature: "You look as though you're missing home. Can you talk about it?"

Returning campers can get homesick too, although their feelings may be tied to missing last year's camp experience more than missing home. Maybe a special camp friend didn't come back or the camper isn't in a preferred cabin or a favorite counselor didn't return.

Homesickness can be a response to a variety of things. Not getting mail can trigger it; not getting "enough" mail or mail from the right people (e.g., boyfriend or girlfriend) can do it. Some kids long for the privacy of their room or miss access to the phone or refrigerator. Some become homesick at times when their parents are typically part of their life (e.g., at meals or bedtime). Usually homesickness reaches a peak by the third or fourth day but, according to Thurber's research (2000), it never really goes away. That's important to remember. It helps to talk with the camper every once in a while and accept homesick feelings as a normal response to missing that which is familiar.

Homesickness can touch anyone — even the nurse!

In most camps it is not appropriate for the camp nurse to call home in the presence of the homesick child. A phone call may come later, but the first step should be to consult the camp director, head counselor, and cabin counselor. To develop strategies to assist the child in the coping process, some nurses conduct a care conference and involve the adults who have a meaningful relationship with the camper. Helpful hints include:

- Keep the camper busy to minimize moments available for thinking about home.
- Enlist the cooperation of other staff. Find out what the child most enjoys and provide an opportunity to spend more time doing it.
- Minimize time the child spends alone by increasing his or her involvement in desirable camp activities.
- Be firm but understanding and supportive when children insist on going home. Behavior of this type is usually a signal that parents should be contacted. They need information about their child's homesickness to partner effectively with camp personnel and, ultimately, help the child. This also helps smooth the situation when homesick letters arrive at home.
- Be sure the camper gets to all meals and activities. Some may try to skip out; often they'll just stay in their cabin. This isn't appropriate because of the supervision risk, the need for social contact, and plain ol' hunger!
- Create a list of suggestions like these that counselors can use when coping with homesick campers.

Diagnosing homesickness can be exasperating. While some children will recognize their feeling and quickly own up to it, others will deny its existence until the day they actually go home. Compounding the issue is the fact that homesickness can make one physically ill. The child can experience nausea, headache, abdominal cramping, shortness of breath, malaise, or vomiting. Or the child might really be ill. Perhaps both are present. This is a time for keen assessment skills!

If at all possible, allow the cabin counselor to initiate the "homesickness cure." The goal is to get a camper so emotionally and physically invested with camp that concerns of home take second place. The cabin group is the prime source of this investment. But keeping the child busy is not the end of concern. Eventually the camper must emotionally confront his or her feelings and learn appropriate coping behaviors. Identifying an adult with whom the camper can talk is a decided asset.

An important step in supporting the growth and development of campers is to include followup for children coping with homesickness. According to Pravda, "At the end of the session, the counselor and nurse should compliment the camper for learning new skills and being able to care for him/herself. Ask the camper to remember the homesick feelings s/he felt when first coming to camp and how they are feeling now that they are leaving. This is how the camper grows, gains insights and learns to cope successfully with separation from home and family" (1995; p. 20).

Chronic Illness

Some campers cope with chronic health problems and come to camp not only for fun activities but also to experience a time in their life when *they* manage their health. Recognizing that there is a knowledgeable adult — the camp nurse — to give help or advice when needed is a boon not only to the children but also to the parents.

Typically, these children send their health form prior to arrival, giving the nurse time to review their case and prepare as needed. While children with chronic concerns need opportunities to be self-reliant, the camp nurse should be prepared to offer occasional boosts

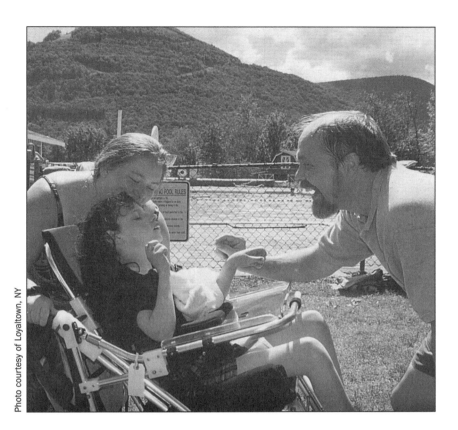

Photo courtesy of Loyaltown, NY

to the camper's level of confidence or intercede if need be. Talk with the parents before the child's arrival; ask if they have questions. Often they will be concerned about the camp staff meeting diet needs, activity or mobility needs, and/or recognizing symptoms that indicate the child needs help. Fill in data gaps so, from a nursing perspective, information is current and thorough.

Consider talking to campers with chronic illnesses within twenty-four hours of arrival to determine their comfort with the camp program. Answer questions they have. Even if the children seem fine, you should talk with them again in a few days because these campers often run on stored energy reserves for the first few days of camp but may need extra rest toward the end of their first week. Their peers recover quickly, but campers with challenges often wear down sooner and have difficulty bouncing back.

Parents of these campers appreciate a call from the nurse, especially when things are going well. These courtesy calls do more than simply reassure anxious parents; they allow the nurse to establish a relationship with the parent that might prove well worthwhile if concerns occur later in the camp season.

Menarche

Most young women are well prepared and ready to experience their first menstrual period. However, not all of them will come to camp with the necessary supplies. The health center should stock emergency supplies until a town trip can be made to purchase items for the girl.

There will probably be a few girls who do not understand what is occurring and may seek your help. Provide the information they need in a tactful and reassuring manner. Anticipate the questions a girl beginning her first menstrual period may have: How often should the pad be changed? Is it okay to swim? How do I take a shower?

Also consider the girl's emotional adjustment to menstruation. For example, this might be a special time for mother and daughter, and the girl may want to call home. Even if the girl is not interested in doing so, the mother might appreciate a call from the nurse.

Behavioral and Emotional Disorders

Children with behavior and/or emotional disorders are usually diagnosed and using a management plan — often one based on medication — before they come to camp. When assessing the child's adaptation to camp in view of their diagnosis, consider the following:

- Is the medication timed appropriate to the camp schedule? Sometimes the medication is a good match for school, but the camp day doesn't end at 3:30 p.m. Some adjustment may be needed.
- Is the medication affected by altitude, hydration status, or other factors that are part of camp yet may not be a component of the home environment?
- Has the camper been on the same medication at the same dose for at least three months before coming to camp? This is often an indicator that a therapeutic blood level has been achieved and/or

that the medication is effective for that child. *Note: Use three months as an indicator, not a definition, of appropriateness.*

- Does the camper have an individualized education plan (IEP) for school? If so, request that a copy be sent to camp. The child's IEP often has good information for activity counselors.
- Does the child have bedtime rituals that might impact cabin life?
- How does fatigue affect this child? This camper might need to be scheduled for an occasional rest hour in the health center.

These and other questions help assess both the child's ability to adjust to camp and the adjustment of others to the child.

Sometimes counseling staff observe unusual behavior from a camper and ask the nurse to check for possible health problems. If you suspect a physical problem, consult with a physician. Some behavior problems, though, are simply a camper's reaction to the stress of being away from home and/or adjusting to camp. Whatever the situation, the camp director is the appropriate person to consult in this situation. Many times this consultation results in a conversation with the parents. Further action is a function of the given situation and beyond the scope of this book.

"Infirmary-itis"

This term refers to the camper who is a chronic complainer and acts as though "going to see the nurse" is an actual camp activity. The usual reason for seeking the nurse's attention is merely that — receiving attention — but homesickness might be at the root and should be treated as we discussed above. Place limits upon this camper while tactfully listening so genuine concerns are not minimized.

Staff Concerns

You'll soon discover that staff members, too, need advice in health and personal matters. Camp staff are typically young adults who are just learning to manage their own health. As a result, they have a variety of questions ranging from how one finds a personal physician to choosing an appropriate analgesic.

Young adults in this situation are extremely vulnerable. They are making health care decisions that may prevail through their lives. It's a good opportunity to provide education, but take care to provide not only correct but culturally sensitive information so they can make informed decisions.

Along with education, you do need to monitor the health of the staff. Camp can be exhausting if one is not getting adequate rest. Slight sore throats and minor headaches lay the groundwork for more serious ailments. Staff should be urged to seek intervention when problems are small. Activities, campers, and other staff feel the effects of someone unable to do their job because of illness.

Eating Concerns

Each summer there seems to be at least one camper or staff member who, because of his or her eating pattern, raises concern about adequate food intake. Often the issue is identified by a counselor who observes that someone "is not eating like they should." The concern is often mentioned at a staff meeting. Be prepared to deal with the issue at that point.

First, establish a reliable data base. Find out what behavior was observed that elicited the remark. Remind staff that people may not feel like eating under certain circumstances (e.g., hot days, when over-tired, having eaten too much candy), nor does it harm a person to miss an occasional meal. It is also important to realize that different people have different eating patterns. Some aren't big eaters; some eat a little bit all day long; some can't seem to get enough at any time. Even acknowledging these situations, you should monitor the reported person's eating pattern; keep a record of what was eaten, the amount, and when. This can be done surreptitiously by you or a counselor. It is important to monitor for at least two days and to include food eaten from the camp's candy store as well as from "care packages."

Along with initial monitoring, consider checking the person's weight to establish a baseline weight using the health center's scale. Compare it to the weight listed on the person's health form, adjusted for date, growth, time of day, and differences between scales.

Assess information in view of the person's eating pattern. For most people, food intake should be adequate to maintain their weight and support their energy needs. Using weight as a key indicator is important. At most camps, the basic concern is that people maintain their weight during their camp stay. This is not to say that people will remain the same weight. The additional activity of camp life will often cause a three- to five-pound weight fluctuation; this should not be a concern.

Some people may want to lose weight during their camp stay. Assuming that they are heavy enough to make this a realistic and healthy goal, an average weight loss of two pounds or less per week is generally acceptable. Sometimes a person may be overambitious and reduce food intake too drastically. It is appropriate to talk to this person and ask her or him to maintain an average loss of two pounds per week while at camp. It is also appropriate — and important — to call parents and discuss concerns with them.

Occasionally, you may be concerned that the behavior indicates anorexia or bulimia. A study completed by Ann W. Moye, Ph.D., licensed psychologist, examined these problems specific to children at camp (1991). In summary, her research indicated that young people may try restricting food intake or throwing up after a meal, but this behavior is typically short-lived and remains subclinical (never amounts to a problem requiring professional intervention) because the child's general good health and limiting ego strength intervene. Nonetheless, it is important to monitor this behavior and to share your observations — not judgements — with the parents.

Moye also observed the counselor's role in reinforcing the social stereotypes that seemingly value physical appearance. In doing her research, Moye was struck by the impact of counselors as role models for campers. This has long been a recognized phenomenon in camping. Moye observed counselors making comments about others: "She should never wear that kind of bathing suit; it looks horrid!" or "Look at those thunder-thighs!" Campers overheard these remarks. From Moye's perspective, such comments reinforced sociological distortions and impressionable campers perceived them as validating those distortions even though the counselors may not have intended them as such. This information is important and well worth discussing with the staff during orientation (and discussing again, if needed).

Psychiatric Concerns

A growing number of people with psychiatric concerns are attending camp. Often these concerns are well-managed as long as the individuals maintain their medication and/or therapeutic regimes.

Occasionally, however, coping patterns break down and questions about a person's continued presence at camp may surface. Consult the camp director. The camp may have access to a psychologist. Recognize the limits of most camps, though. They are not designed as therapeutic programs.

Ask if the person participates in a form of talk therapy: individual or group. Note the name of the therapist in case concerns arise over time.

Note that some people with psychiatric concerns find it difficult to live in their cabins. Many have their own room at home or share that room with one other person. Coping with the ambient noise of ten to twelve people can be wearing and coping reserves may fatigue after a few days. Consequently, you should talk with these individuals after three or four days to ask how things are going. Note signs of fatigue: circles under their eyes, increased sensitivity, angry outbursts. Be prepared to intervene. Sometimes simple devices — such as providing earphones so they can listen to music while falling asleep — may be all that's needed to help them cope.

Sometimes a camper or staff member is not able to remain safe or threatens the safety of others. Safety is the bottom line at most camps. If an individual is causing harm to him- or herself or others, the camp director must be notified. Do not attempt to resolve this without input from the director.

CHAPTER 13

Finishing Touches

When You're the Nurse
and Your Child Is a Camper

Some nurses take a camp nurse position when their child is ready for camp. They are then in the dual roles of employee and parent. This combination should be thoroughly thought through. It often requires adaptation from both the parent and the child. The camp wants a nurse who can effectively work the job. The camp does not want a parent who thinks working as a camp nurse will provide all kinds of time for a unique experience focusing on the parent-child bond. It usually won't. The child will have a camper experience; the nurse needs to focus on the camp nurse's job.

Going to camp together is fine for many parent-child dyads. The child comfortably transitions to viewing the counseling staff as any other camper would; there is no need to constantly touch base with the parent for reassurance. And the nurse is able to move the child into the cabin and leave the parenting role until the end of season (with the occasional hug sprinkled into mealtimes perhaps).

For others, it may be more of a struggle. For example, the first few days of working as a camp nurse are often the busiest and most wor-

159

risome. The nurse is adjusting to the new position just as the camper adjusts to being a camper. Separation from home might be slightly easier for a child whose parent is on site, but the camper needs to realize, before camp starts, that Mom or Dad has a very busy job and will not be readily available. The child eats with the cabin and not the parent. It is a very wise nurse who realistically discusses camp life with the child before going to camp. The nurse and child will have a much more positive camp experience.

Separation from home may also have a pull on the parent. Things that you take for granted — access to favorite food, the ability to go places at almost any time, availability of phones to call friends, one's bed — give way to camp benefits: not having to cook, saving gas money, being outdoors. Sometimes those benefits pale during the flurry of Opening Day when your life is quite busy. Even mealtimes can be impacted because you may be extremely busy dispensing medication and checking with other campers and staff.

When you are walking about camp, you certainly can greet and visit with your child but as a part of visiting with all the campers in the group. Do not interrupt a camp activity to visit with your child; just wave to everyone and visit later. As the nurse, you will be busy and there won't be much time to write your child. It is good to prepare some cards, comics, or packages before leaving for camp and have a relative or friend mail them to your child. Receiving mail is very important to campers — even if they are the nurse's kids!

Sometimes concern about parent-child dyads will exist within the staff. Some staff, especially counselors, may feel that having a parent on staff means they need to treat the camper differently. Use staff orientation or a staff meeting to emphasize that you want your child to be treated like a regular camper and you are their camp nurse, not parent-in-residence.

Even though you and your child are at the same camp, the child will have a very different experience from you. The stories that come home may make you wonder if you actually were at the same place! This is a positive for both of you.

Partnering with Parents

Camps are for campers. Nonetheless, campers' parents should be involved with health care concerns and have an active role in decision making for their campers. The camp physician will focus on the camper's injury or illness; the camp nurse needs to remember to connect with the parents. Discuss parent contact with the camp director, not only when to call parents but also how to document both conversations and unsuccessful attempts to reach parents. Be sensitive to issues surrounding custodial parent rights, legal guardians, and divorce situations, and follow the camp director's guidance.

Sometimes parents aren't home when calls are placed. A growing number have answering machines that can be accessed remotely. In other words, they want the camp to leave a message. The need to do this is magnified by the prevalence of call-identification devices. It's harrowing for a parent to come home, note that the camp's number shows on their machine, but find no message! Consequently, before placing a call home, consider the message you might leave.

Sometimes parents assume that the camp nurse is familiar with their child's overall camp adjustment. So another tip is to ask the camp director "Is there anything I should know about this camper?" before placing a parental call. Is the camper receiving mail, participating in activities, eating normally? This information is extremely important, especially if the camper has had some earlier problem at camp and the parents have previously been contacted. Be prepared for a parent to ask, "How does my child like camp? He wrote home you had spaghetti three nights in a row." Remember: calls to parents are also public relations for the camp.

The Health Center Is the Nurse's Camp Home

Enjoy the health center. Take ownership and make the facility homey. Bring a colorful bedspread, a radio, and/or a CD player. Decorate the walls. Campers are very creative and love to draw and paint. Most of all, they enjoy seeing their work displayed. Have them draw pictures with a health theme: Have you had your 8 Glasses of Water today? DRINK! DRINK! DRINK! Avoid this Plant! Wash Your Hands!

Consider the Health Center Budget

Most camps, like the rest of the world, are under budget constraints. Take this into consideration when setting up the health center. Rather than buy, first look around camp for items that can be appropriated for health center needs. For example, the ice cream tubs make perfect "throw up" containers or individual wastebaskets for tissues. Ask the arts and crafts director for poster board, paint, lanyard material, yarn, or other supplies for ill campers. Ask the local pharmacist to save last year's PDR for camp. Ask the camp physician or your own personal physician for supplies. Some doctors will supply a case of nonlatex gloves, tongue blades, etc. The dentist might donate toothbrushes or toothpaste, and the orthodontist could provide wax for braces and rubber bands. "Ask and you shall receive!"

A Short History of Camp Nursing

Camp nursing is still a work in progress. Literature is sparse; research is even rarer. But health services have long been a part of organized camping. Reference to the topic first appeared in connection with Joseph Rothrock's camp for "weakly boys," the Mountain School of Physical Culture in Luzerne, Pennsylvania. Founded in 1876 by Rothrock, a physician, the camp was designed to boost the health of frail boys by having them live outdoors while continuing their education (Eells, 1986; Meier and Mitchell, 1993). Since organized camping generally recognizes its start with the Gunnery in 1861, the appearance of Rothrock's camp shortly thereafter indicates the value placed on nature as a healing element, especially for children.

That value continues today. Although literature is not abundant, anecdotal history bears testimony to the presence of the camp nurse, and ACA Standards reflect continued interest in the health of campers and staff. Nursing's influence, however, has only recently been recognized in any significant way.

During the 1960s, Jeanne Otto, RN, took her children to camp. "Through eight summers of practice, I researched, questioned, observed and gathered data, thus learning what I needed to know. . . . I realized that all camp nurses experience similar difficulties, especially in their initial experience. . . . In 1975, as an offering of the North-eastern University Department of Continuing Education, I initiated a pre-camp workshop for camp nurses" (Otto, 1980; Foreword). Jeanne also used her camp nursing experience in research that later became her master thesis: "There was no documentation of the camp nurse role. Thus evolved this study" (Otto, 1980; Foreword).

Soon Jeanne was teaching nursing and had added a couple of master's degrees to her vitae. She continued to write. Word of mouth passed along the message that Jeanne would send you a letter once, maybe twice a year if you sent her $10. Many of us did that. We were on Jeanne's mailing list forever. It was a good investment, one which marked the start of the camp nurse network.

While Jeanne was developing her ideas, Mary Lou Hemessley, RN, wrote the *Handbook for Camp Nurses and Other Camp Health Workers* in 1973. Soon after, the American Nurses' Association in cooperation with the Washington State Nurses Association published the *Standards for Nursing Services in Camp Settings* (1978).

Meanwhile, Louise Czupryna, RN, instructor at the University of Southern Maine School of Nursing, began teaching "Health Care in the Camp Setting" and developed one of the earliest reference lists for camp nursing. There were not many citations by camp nurses and that precious few came predominantly from nurses at special needs camps who wrote anecdotally of their experience. But there were also some glittering selections from nurses who continue to be active in camp nursing today:

- Mary Casey wrote *The Nurse and the Health Program in Camp* in 1984.
- Louise Czupryna published "Primary Prevention in the Camp Setting" in *Maternal Child Nursing*, 1984.
- Myra Pravda published "The Camp Health Program and Staff Orientation" in *Pediatric Nursing*, 1988, and followed it with her book, *Off to Camp!* in 1990.

1990 was a hallmark year for camp nursing. The American Camping Association held its national conference in Boston that February and, seizing an opportunity, Jeanne Otto wrote to everyone on her mailing list announcing the first "camp nurse meeting."

In essence, Jeanne also announced her retirement from teaching and, with it, the retirement of her famous letter "unless someone does something about it."

Someone did. In fact, thirteen "someones" responded. On February 24, 1990, thirteen camp nurses attended the first of what came to be called the Association of Camp Nurses' Conference. After presentations about AIDS and Lyme disease, Jeanne convened a business meeting that resulted in formation of ACN's first Board of Directors and election of the first president. The first action was to change the dues structure to a $10 annual fee. That was closely followed by articulating a focus for the Association: "to collect and disseminate camp nursing information, advocate for the practice area, and affiliate with professional nursing as well as the camping profession" (Erceg, 1990).

ACN's First Board of Directors

Nancy Baver, Ely, MN
Tricia Barr, Hanover, NH
Diane Cohen, Framingham, MA
Sherri Ebner, Harwinton, CT
Linda Ebner Erceg, Bemidji, MN
Margaret Ellis, Wiscasset, ME
Lynn Greene, Natick, MA
Kathleen Leon, Glendale, CA
Jeanne Otto, Cambridge, MA
Myra Pravda, Cincinnati, OH
Martha Schelling, Naples, FL
Rosalie Sullivan, Medford, MA
Beth Thomson, No-Reading, MA

Meanwhile, the College of Nurses of Ontario (Canada) published *Camp Nursing Guidelines for RNs and RNAs* (1990) and Ontario's Camp Healthcare Committee, led by nurses Mary Casey and Pearl Bell, expanded its role. On a grimmer note, ANA ceased publication of its *Standards for Nursing Services in Camp Settings* because "there hasn't been enough demand for the piece" (personal communication; October, 1990).

Nonetheless, camp nursing continued to move forward. Kay Totten, RN, and Carolyn Hudgens, RN, began teaching college courses at Lewis Clark State College and University of Iowa, respectively, about camp nursing. ACN was incorporated in 1994, the same year that Kris Lishner taught her summer course, "Role Development in Child Health Promotion in Nontraditional Settings," and offered graduate credit through Washington State University for nursing study at camp. This was rapidly followed by the publication of her book, *Creating a Healthy Camp Community: A Nurse's Role*. ACN expanded its newsletter to four issues a year and, with the Fall 1995 issue, established *CompassPoint*.

Camp-nurse educational opportunities expanded from the three available in 1990 to the fourteen of 2001. Annual education events have taken place since Boston's 1990 event. These culminated with 1999's International Camp Health Conference. The annual Camp Nurse Symposium, held in the Chicago area each spring, is now established as the only annual event designed for experienced camp nurses; it continues to draw more and more nurses. The *Standards and Scope of Camp Nursing Practice*, recently approved by ACN members, is now available. And both a Web site (www.campnurse.org) and an online Camp Nurse discussion group support the growing number of nurses who have discovered camp nursing as their practice niche.

Yet there's so much more to be done. Camps continue to need nurses. Research must be started and more literature developed. The practice is in its infancy but it's also a sparkling practice, one of the few where a nurse can truly practice nursing, experience the autonomy of a professional role, and make a difference in the lives of children, youth, and young adults.

The things that have been accomplished were done by nurses who cared about kids and camp. There are many, but our camps need many more. Won't you join us?

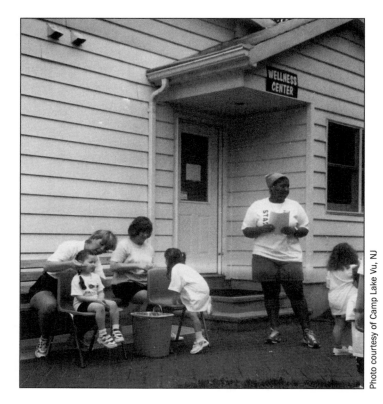

Photo courtesy of Camp Lake Vu, NJ

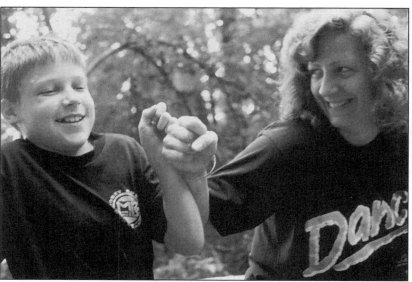

Photo courtesy of Camp Easter Seals, VA

References and Resources

■ References

American Camping Association (1998). *Accreditation Standards for Camp Programs and Services.* Martinsville, IN: American Camping Association.

American Camping Association (2001). *How to Choose a Camp.* http://www.ACAcamps.org/media/choose.htm [26 February 2001].

Arizona Department of Health Services (1998). *Physician's Guide to Dental Emergencies.* Oakland, CA: Dental Health Foundation.

Association of Camp Nurses (2001). *The Standards and Scope of Camp Nursing Practice.* Bemidji, MN: Association of Camp Nurses.

Backer, H., Bowman, W., Paton, B., Steele, P. and Thygerson, A. (1998). *Wilderness First Aid.* Sudbury, MA: Jones and Bartlett.

Black, J. and Matassarin-Jacobs, E. (1997). *Medical-Surgical Nursing.* Philadelphia: Saunders.

Casey, M. (1997). *Camp Health Care.* Waterloo, ON: Conestoga Printing.

Chin, J., ed. (2000). *Control of Communicable Diseases Manual.* Washington, DC: American Public Health Association.

College of Nurses of Ontario. (1990). *Camp Nursing Guidelines for RNs and RNAs.* Toronto: College of Nurses of Ontario.

Coutellier, C. and Henchey, K. (2000). *Camp Is for the Camper.* Martinsville, IN: American Camping Association.

Crane, A. (2000). "Five Rookie Mistakes and Five Lessons Learned." *CompassPoint* 10 (3), pp. 4–6.

Czupryna, L. (1984). "Primary Prevention in the Camp Setting." *Maternal Child Nursing* 9 (3), pp. 197–199.

Eells, E. (1986). *History of Organized Camping: The First 100 years.* Martinsville, IN: American Camping Association.

Erceg, L. (1990). "ACN Conference Outcomes." *Camp Nurse Newsletter*, Spring 1990, p. 3. Available from Association of Camp Nurses, Bemidji, MN.

Erceg, L. (1996). "Probing Injury-Illness Information of the Concordia Language Villages, 1991–1995." Master's thesis, University of North Dakota, Grand Forks, ND.

Erceg, L. (1999a). "Common Ground: Camp Health Services Come of Age." Paper presented at the Association of Camp Nurses' International Camp Health Conference, Bemidji, MN.

Erceg, L. (1999b). "Managing Camp Health and Safety. Paper presented at the Association of Camp Nurses' International Camp Health Conference, Bemidji, MN.

Forgey, W., ed. (2001). Practice Guidelines for Wilderness Emergency Care. Guilford, CT: Globe Pequot Press.

Hamlessley, M. (1977). *Handbook for Camp Nurses and Other Camp Health Workers.* New York: Tiresias Press.

Hauser, S. (1996). *Nature's Revenge.* New York: Lyons and Burford.

Lishner, K. and Busch, K. (1994). "Safe Delivery of Medications to Children in Summer Camps." *Pediatric Nursing* 20 (3), pp. 249–253.

Lishner, K. M. and Bruya, M. A. (1994). *Creating a Healthy Camp Community: A Nurse's Role.* Martinsville, IN: American Camping Association.

Meier, J. and Mitchell, A .V. (1993). *Camp Counseling.* Madison, WI: Brown and Benchmark.

Neinstein, L. (1996). *Adolescent Health Care: A Practical Guide.* Baltimore: Williams and Wilkins.

Otto, J. (1980). *Profile of the Camp Nurse in New England.* Chicago: Fund for the Advancement of Camping.

Pravda, M. (1988). "The Camp Health Program and Staff Orientation." *Pediatric Nursing* 14 (3), pp. 184–186.

Pravda, M. (1990). *Off to Camp!.* Cincinnati, OH: JSP Publishing.

Pravda, M. (1995). "Homesickness: Dispelling the Myths." *Camping Magazine,* 67 (4), pp. 18–20.

Rudolf, M. C., Alario, A. J., Youth, B. and Riggs, S. (1993). "Self-Medication in Childhood: Observations at a Residential Summer Camp." *Pediatrics,* 91, pp. 1182–1184.

Thurber, C. (2000). *The Summer Camp Handbook.* Los Angeles: Perspective Publishing.

Thygerson, A. (2001). *First Aid and CPR.* Boston: Jones and Bartlett.

■ Resources

American Camping Association
5000 State Road 67 North, Martinsville, IN 46151-7902.
Phone: 800-428-2267.
www.ACAcamps.org
Guide to ACA-Accredited Camps; sponsors conferences; many resources online and in ACA Bookstore.

Association of Camp Nurses
8504 Thorsonveien N.E., Bemidji, MN 56601.
Phone: 218-586-2633.
www.campnurse.org
CompassPoint; sponsors conferences; promotes camp nurse networking.

Center for Disease Control
1600 Clifton Road, N.E., Atlanta, GA 30333.
Phone: 800-311-3435.
www.cdc.gov
Resource for specific illnesses, traveler information, and public health alerts.

Food Allergy Network
10400 Eaton Place, Suite 107, Fairfax, VA 22030.
Phone: 800-929-4040.
www.foodallergy.org
Camp Guide to Managing Severe Allergic Reactions; source of EpiPen trainers; recipes.

Wilderness Medical Society
3595 East Fountain Boulevard., Colorado Springs, CO 80910.
Phone: 719-572-9255.
www.wms.org
Practice Guidelines for Wilderness Emergency Care; *Wilderness and Environmental Medicine*; slide sets; memberships available.

APPENDIX A

Suggestions for Camp First Aid Kits

■ **Contents for In-Camp Kits** *(assumes camp nurse is available)*

- Adhesive tape
- Assorted adhesive strip bandages
- Black pen, indelible black marker
- CPR mask
- Disposable gloves (vinyl, not latex)
- Elastic wrap (3" or 4")
- Scissors
- Sealable plastic bag for infectious waste
- Skin antiseptic — wipes or plastic squeeze bottle
- Small notebook
- Sterile dressings, individually packaged
- Triangular bandage(s)
- Tweezers

■ **Additions to First Aid Kits in Specialized Areas**

- **Waterfront:** plastic airways, backboard, sunscreen (30 SPF minimum), insect repellent
- **Kitchen:** finger cots, 4-tailed knuckle bandages, Rx Silvadene
- **Maintenance:** instant ice packs, sunscreen (30 SPF minimum), insect repellent, poison ivy barrier cream, eye-flushing solution
- **Horseback riding:** instant ice packs, sunscreen (30 SPF minimum), insect repellent
- **Housekeeping:** instant ice packs, finger cots, eye shield and flushing solution

■ **Items That Should NOT Be in Camp First Aid Kits**

- **Aerosol containers:** These items can overheat in the sun and increase the potential for discharge or harm.
- **Glass containers:** Potential for breakage and consequent contamination of other items.
- **Medications:** These are inappropriate for most first aid kits. If added — for example, Silvadene in the kitchen's kit — people using the kit should be taught about the medication's use and when the situation is no longer in the domain of first aid and must be referred to the camp nurse.

■ Suggested Additional Items for Kits Used in Out-of-Camp Settings

- Ace bandages, 3" or 4" and 6"
- Copy of participant health forms and permission-to-treat statements
- Emergency contact numbers
- Emergency meds: epinephrine, analgesics, antihistamines; see note above
- Individual medications (i.e., daily meds needed by participants); see note above
- Instant ice packs (disposable)
- Mechanism for purifying water
- Moleskin
- Sunblock, insect repellent
- Temperature-taking device
- Triangular bandages
- Steri-strips
- Tweezers
- Waterproof storage container for kit

APPENDIX B
Sample Protocol for Screening

The person responsible for screening must have in hand the individual's health history. It should be signed by parent, guardian, or adult responsible for the individual, preferably within six months prior to the screening. Screening shall occur within twenty-four hours of an individual's arrival at camp.

When screening a person, identify any observable evidence of illness, disability, or communicable disease. Review the health history and check it for appropriate signature. Special attention should be noted for (1) current medications and/or treatment procedures, (2) dietary restrictions, (3) allergies, and (4) physical limitations. All important items must be recorded on the individual's health record and a screening note completed per camp protocol.

Additionally, these questions must be asked of each person during the screening process and their response recorded:

a. Are you currently taking any medication not already noted on your health form?
b. Have you been exposed to a communicable disease within the past three weeks?
c. Are you ill or injured now?
d. Is there anything to change or add to the health form that isn't already on it?

Individuals who come to camp with evidence of illness, communicable disease, or disability should be evaluated by a licensed physician and, based on the outcome of the evaluation, a decision made about the individual's readiness to participate at camp.

APPENDIX C

Sample Diet Form for Camp Kitchen

Name of Person	Vegetarian				Food Allergy Information		
	Semi	Pesco	Lacto Ovo	Vegan	Allergen	Intol.	Needs Epi

Other Diet Information	
Name of Person	Dietary Note, Explanation

APPENDIX D

Suggested Interview for Person with Asthma

Client's Name _____   □ Camper □ Staff Member

Date of Interview _____

About Triggers

What triggers your asthma?   Gather details about the triggers, including
□ Exercise   things cabin and activity staff should be told.
□ Fatigue
□ Dehydration   _____
□ Stress
□ Food Item   _____
□ Smoke
□ Respiratory infections/common cold
□ Allergen _____
□ Other   _____

Using a Peak Flow Meter

We recommend using a peak flow meter as a way to monitor your asthma
and note signs of a potential flare before it is well-established.

When does this person take peak flow readings?
□ Breakfast □ Lunch □ Supper □ Bedtime □ Other _____

Routine peak flow reading for this person (green range) _____

Caution range (yellow) _____

What is done if the peak flow reading drops to the caution/yellow range?

_____

Danger range (red zone) _____

What is done if peak flow reading drops to the danger/red zone? _____

_____

About Medications

These medications are used daily to manage this person's asthma.

Medication Name	Dose Given	When	Reason for Using This Med

These medications are taken "as needed" to prevent an asthma flare.

Medication Name	Dose Given	When	Reason for Using This Med

These medications are used when the person's asthma flares

Medication Name	Dose to Be Given	At What Point Should This Be Used?	What Effect Should Be Expected and How Quickly?

Nebulizer Treatment and Use

Did you bring a nebulizer to camp? .... □ Yes □ No

If yes, do you know when you need your nebulizer? .... □ Yes □ No

What medication is used via nebulizer? _____

When there are questions about your asthma, who should we contact?

Name _____ Phone _____

Name _____ Phone _____

At what point should we notify someone else about an asthma flare and who should be told?

_____

_____

_____

At what point should you be taken to a physician/emergency room?

_____

_____

_____

APPENDIX E
Suggested Interview for Person with Diabetes

Client's Name _____   □ Camper   □ Staff Member

Date of Interview _____

About Your Routine Diabetes Care

□ When do you check your blood sugar (BS)? _____

□ What is your usual range of BS readings? _____

□ When (at what time) do you regularly inject insulin? _____

What type is used and how many units? _____

□ In addition to meals, describe your pattern for snacks (time, what you eat, etc.).

_____

_____

_____

□ If a question about diabetes management arises, who do we call? At what number?

_____

_____

□ Other people may have questions about your diabetes. Are you comfortable talking about it?   □ Yes   □ No   If yes, what would you tell them?

_____

_____

_____

About Your Reaction When Your Blood Sugar Is Low

□ If your BS gets low, what signs or behaviors should we expect?

_____

_____

_____

□ If you get low, what should we do? _____

- ☐ Do certain stressors tend to drop your BS? What are they?

- ☐ When was your last low blood sugar reaction? _____

  How often do you have low reactions? _____

- ☐ Have you ever had a severely low blood sugar reaction (seizure, loss of consciousness)? ☐ No ☐ Yes   If yes, what happened?

Additional Information

- ☐ If your blood sugar is running high, what signs or behaviors would we see and what do you want us/me to do?

- ☐ Who do you want us to notify if you have a reaction? (Get appropriate phone/fax numbers.)

- ☐ Name of your diabetes educator _____
  Phone _____
- ☐ What else would you like us to know?

Sample Daily Medication Record (DMR)

Camp Anywhere U.S.A.
Daily Medication Record

Camp Session Dates: __2-13 July 2001__

☐ Staff DMR   ☑ Camper DMR

Name and Medication Order	Hr	Jul 2 M	Jul 3 T	Jul 4 W	Jul 5 Th	Jul 6 F	Jul 7 S	Jul 8 Sn	Jul 9 M	Jul 10 T	Jul 11 W	Jul 12 Th	Jul 13 F
Puddlehopper, Nellie													
• Seldane 60 mg qD for allergy	8a	→	LEE	LEE	LEE	LEE	LEE	LEE	LEE	LEE	LEE	LEE	LEE
Swattum, Bugsy	8a	→	LEE	LEE	LEE								
• Pen-VeeK 125 mg TID	12	→	LEE	LEE	LEE	DC'ed - ℛ × Completed							
for Otitis media	6p	LEE	LEE	LEE	LEE								
Healthwise, Inertia													
• Multi-Vit i qD per parent	8a	→	LEE	LEE	LEE	LEE	LEE	LEE	○	LEE	LEE	LEE	Home
We-no-Wheeze, Ebenezer	8a	→	self	self	self	self	self	self	self	self	self	self	Home
• Protentil 1-2 puffs BID	8p	self	self	self	self	self	self	self	self	self	self	self	
Rashman, Scratch	8a	———————————→								LEE	LEE	LEE	Home
• Bactroban BID to area	8p	———————————→								LEE	LEE	LEE	LEE

Medication dispensed and recorded by:

Name: __Linda Ebner Erceg__ Initial: _LEE_ Credential: _ℛℕ_

Name: _____ Initial: _____ Credential: _____

Name: _____ Initial: _____ Credential: _____

APPENDIX G
Recipes for the Health Center

- **Saline Gargle for Sore Throats.** Dissolve 4 tablespoons of salt in 1 gallon of water. Mix a fresh solution each day and keep at room temperature in a self-dispensing, covered container for use as needed.
- **Cold Packs.** Dampen paper toweling with water and fold it to fit inside a sealable baggie; then freeze it. Use as needed with appropriate thermal barrier.
- **Slush Packs.** *(Caution: Assess your clients! Will campers drink this?)* Mix 1 tablespoon of isopropyl alcohol in 1 cup of water. Add blue food coloring to tint the mixture "ice blue" and pour into a freezer-quality sealable baggie; freeze. The mixture becomes a slurry consistency that molds to body parts (e.g., ankle, knee). After use, wipe with bacteriostatic wipe and refreeze.

  Make several to store in the kitchen's big freezer. The packs are handy when several people get stung at the same time! Be sure to store them in a container clearly marked "Health Center Use Only" and tell clients *not* to drink the liquid. Variation: Dampen a washcloth with the water and alcohol mixture.
- **Baking Soda Paste for Stings.** Put about 1 tablespoon of baking soda in a medicine cup. Carefully add a bit of water and stir to the consistency of Elmer's Glue. Dollop the mixture directly onto a sting area after the stinger has been removed to cool and relieve discomfort. Instruct the client to apply more as needed. The water evaporates, leaving a dry, caked pile of baking soda that is easily removed with gentle rubbing or running water.

> **Practice Hint:**
> Keep a few med cups with baking soda in a handy place and a dropper bottle of water nearby. You can then quickly mix the paste when needed.

- **Sanitizing Solution.** Mix 1 tablespoon bleach in 3 quarts of water. This makes a 200 parts per million sanitizing solution (the minimum is 100 parts per million) that is used to disinfect surfaces (e.g., beds, counter tops, floors). The solution deteriorates given time and with exposure to protein (e.g., bacteria); consequently, it is advisable to mix a new batch each day.

- **Individual Ice Cubes.** Make single ice cubes by filling medicine cups with water and placing them in the freezer. They freeze quickly, are easy to grab, and make great "bug bite coolers" or ice-rub devices. They're also great to cool iced tea!

Index

records. *See* health records
referrals to out-of-camp providers, 73
refilling prescriptions, 99
refrigeration, 32
regulations for medication management, 90
repairs, health center, 26
reports, final, 58
required reading, prior to camp, 21–22
rescue inhalers, 91
residential camps, 16
resources, 169
Rest Hour, 61
RICE (rest, ice, compression, elevation), injuries and, 105
ringworm, 136
Rothrock, Joseph, 162
Rudolf, Alario, Youth, and Riggs, self-management and, 89

S

salary information, 20
saline gargle solution, 183
sanitation
  food service, 76
  health center, 66–67
  table setting, 30
  Walk-around and, 52–53
sanitizing solution recipe, 67, 183–184
scheduling
  office hours and, 60–62
  special events and, 53–55
screening, 13
  communicable diseases and, 107–108
  how/where, 42–45
  Opening Day, 37–45
  prescreen health forms, 39
  protocol suggestion, 173
  recordkeeping, 85
  sample procedure, 43–45
  staff, 38
    precamp, 26
security
  forms, 32
  medications, 32, 90–92
  records, 32
seizure disorders, counselors and, 41
self-care techniques, 112–113

self-designed recordkeeping systems, 84
self-managing medication, 87–88
  nurse's responsibility, 92
  Rudolf, Alario, Youth, and Riggs and, 89
separation anxiety, 149–152
sessions
  health team transition, 58
  last day, 57–58
  medications, 55
  multiple, 55–57
  paperwork, 55
severe weather, 30
sharps container, 64
shock, 136–137
showers, Walk-around and, 53
sick call, 51. *See also* office hours
sleep disorders, counselors and, 41
slivers/splinters, 114, 138
slush packs, 183
sore throats, 113, 138–139
  saline gargle, 183
special events, 53–55
special needs camps, 17
special needs diets, 40
splinters, 114, 138
sprains, 139–140
staff, 18. *See also* healthcare staff
  care of, vs. campers, 59–60
  emotional health, 155–156
  health orientation, 24, 27–30
  health screening, 26
  health screenings, 38
  interview information, 20
  medication management, 92
  nurse's relationship, 22–23
staff-only office hours, 61
staff orientation. *See* precamp
standard precautions, 103
The Standards and Scope of Camp Nursing Practice, 16, 18, 60, 165
Standards for Nursing Services in Camp Settings, 164
standing orders, 112
state regulations for medications, 27
stings, 114
  baking soda paste, 183
stitches, 69
stock medications, 13
stomach flu, 117